Dear Scarlet

Dear Scarlet

THE STORY OF MY POSTPARTUM DEPRESSION

Teresa Wong

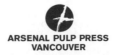

ARSENAL PULP PRESS
VANCOUVER

ARSENAL PULP PRESS
Suite 202 – 211 East Georgia St.
Vancouver, BC V6A 1Z6
Canada
arsenalpulp.com

The publisher gratefully acknowledges the support of the Canada Council for the Arts and the British Columbia Arts Council for its publishing program, and the Government of Canada, and the Government of British Columbia (through the Book Publishing Tax Credit Program), for its publishing activities.

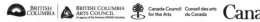

British Columbia | British Columbia Arts Council An agency of the Province of British Columbia | Canada Council for the Arts Conseil des arts du Canada | Canadä

Arsenal Pulp Press acknowledges the xʷməθkʷəy̓əm (Musqueam), Sḵwx̱wú7mesh (Squamish), and səl̓ilwətaʔɬ (Tsleil-Waututh) Nations, speakers of Hul'q'umi'num'/Halq'eméylem/hən̓q̓əmin̓əm̓ and custodians of the traditional, ancestral, and unceded territories where our office is located. We pay respect to their histories, traditions, and continuous living cultures and commit to accountability, respectful relations, and friendship.

Edited by Shirarose Wilensky
Proofread by Alison Strobel

Printed and bound in Canada

Library and Archives Canada Cataloguing in Publication:
Wong, Teresa, 1976-, author
Dear Scarlet : the story of my postpartum depression / Teresa Wong.
Issued in print and electronic formats.
ISBN 978-1-55152-765-9 (softcover).—ISBN 978-1-55152-766-6 (PDF)
1. Wong, Teresa, 1976- —Comic books, strips, etc. 2. Wong, Teresa, 1976- —Health—Comic books, strips, etc. 3. Postpartum depression—Comic books, strips, etc. 4. Postpartum depression—Patients—Canada—Biography—Comic books, strips, etc. 5. Mothers—Canada—Biography—Comic books, strips, etc. 6. Motherhood—Comic books, strips, etc. 7.Autobiographical comics. I. Title.
RG852.W66 2019 362.1987'60092 C2018-906210-X
C2018-906211-8

This is a love letter
to my three children
and my mother.

Dear Scarlet

The other day, you told me that when you grow up, you want to be a mommy.

I said you could be anything you wanted...
ARTIST
DOCTOR
TEACHER
and ALSO be a mommy.

But you were adamant about it.
MOMMY

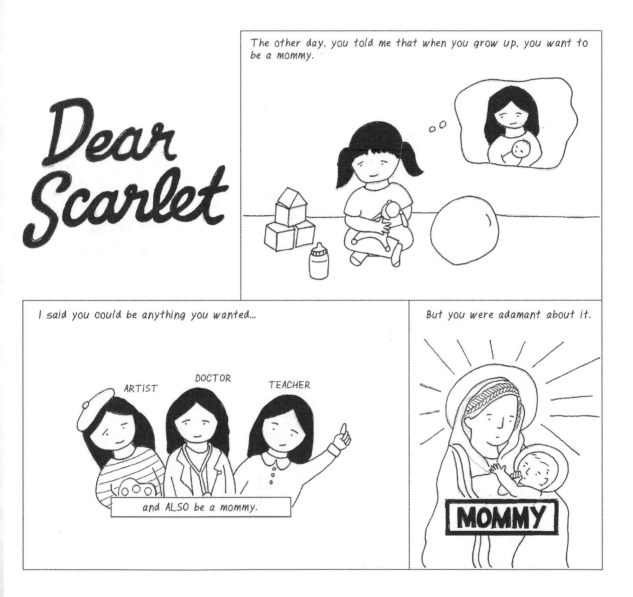

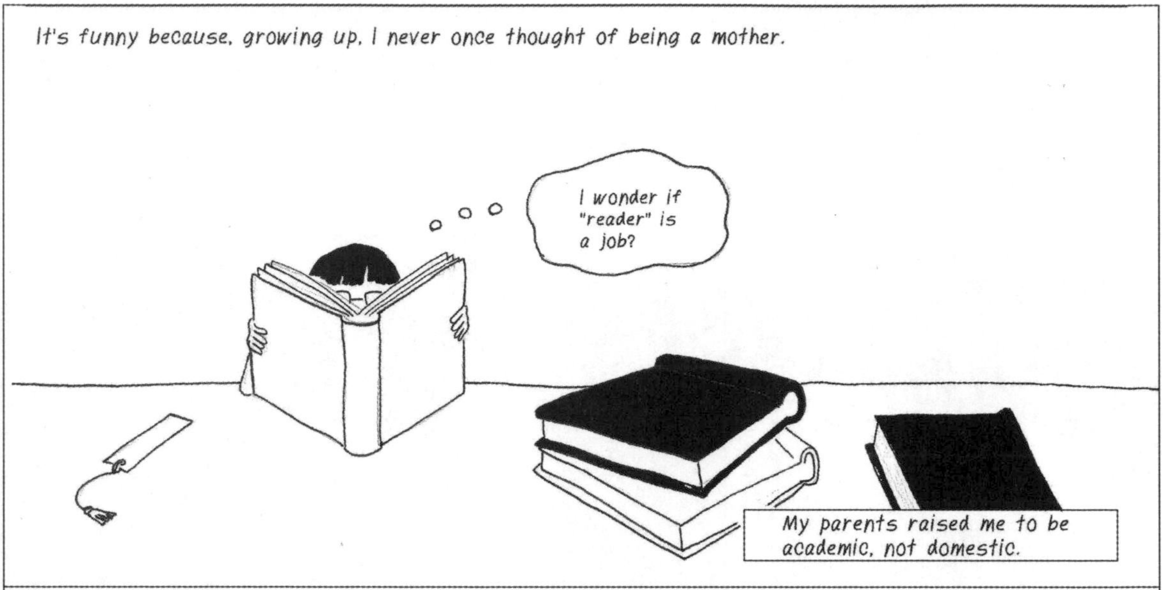
It's funny because, growing up, I never once thought of being a mother.
I wonder if "reader" is a job?
My parents raised me to be academic, not domestic.

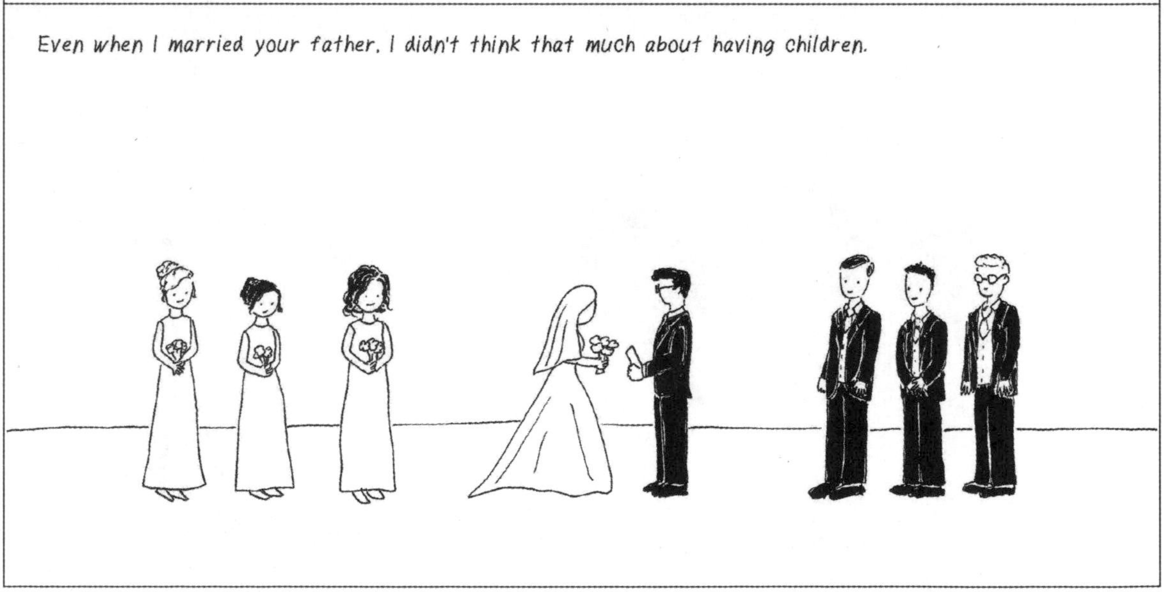
Even when I married your father, I didn't think that much about having children.

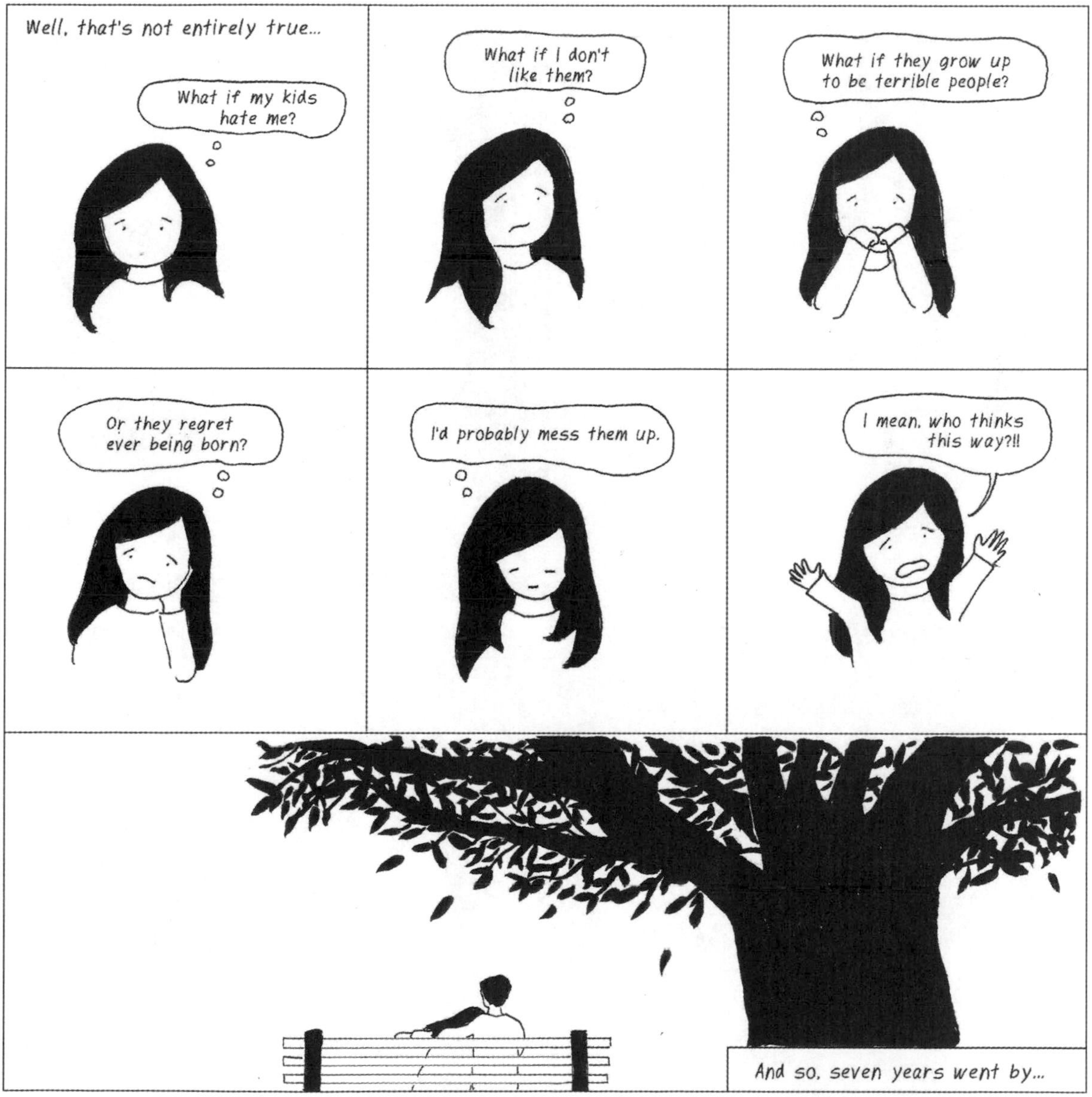
Well, that's not entirely true...
What if my kids hate me?
What if I don't like them?
What if they grow up to be terrible people?
Or they regret ever being born?
I'd probably mess them up.
I mean, who thinks this way?!!
And so, seven years went by...

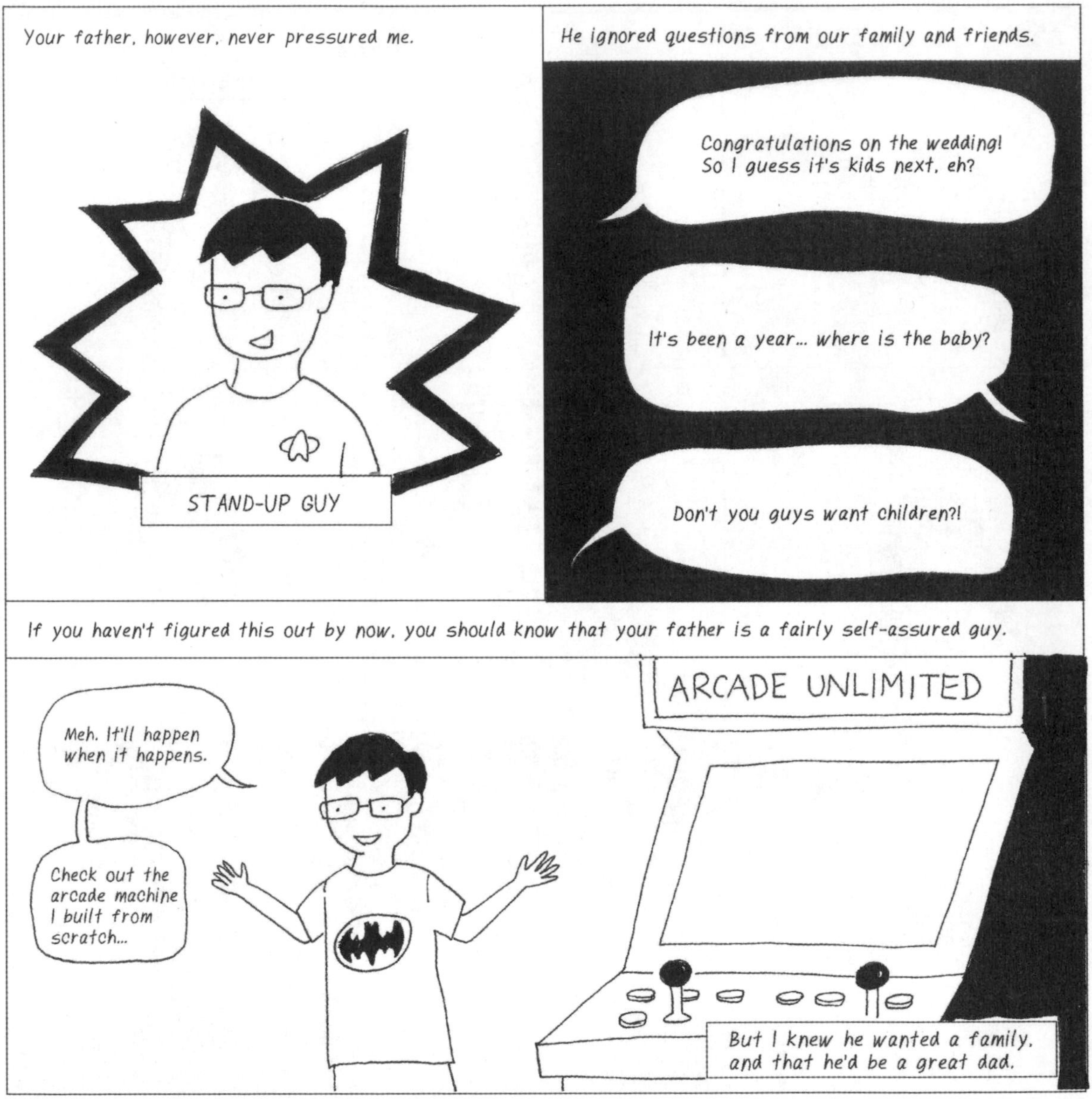
Your father, however, never pressured me.
STAND-UP GUY
He ignored questions from our family and friends.
Congratulations on the wedding! So I guess it's kids next, eh?
It's been a year... where is the baby?
Don't you guys want children?!
If you haven't figured this out by now, you should know that your father is a fairly self-assured guy.
Meh. It'll happen when it happens.
Check out the arcade machine I built from scratch...
ARCADE UNLIMITED
But I knew he wanted a family, and that he'd be a great dad.

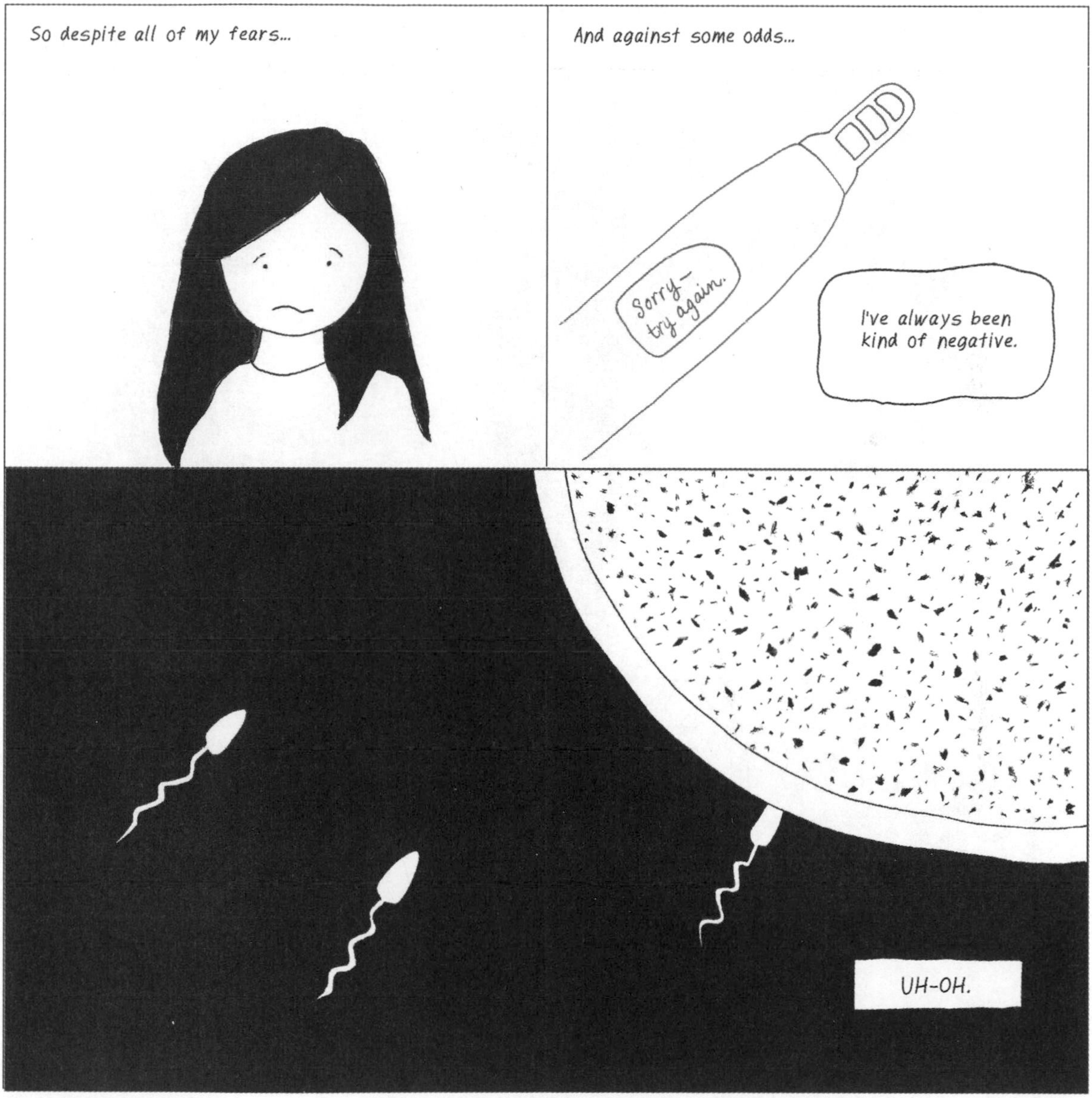
So despite all of my fears...
And against some odds...
Sorry— try again.
I've always been kind of negative.
UH-OH.

MY PREGNANCY

* NOT FOR THE FAINT OF HEART *

How can I vomit so much and still be alive?
How can I be so tired and still be alive?
Please, kill me now.

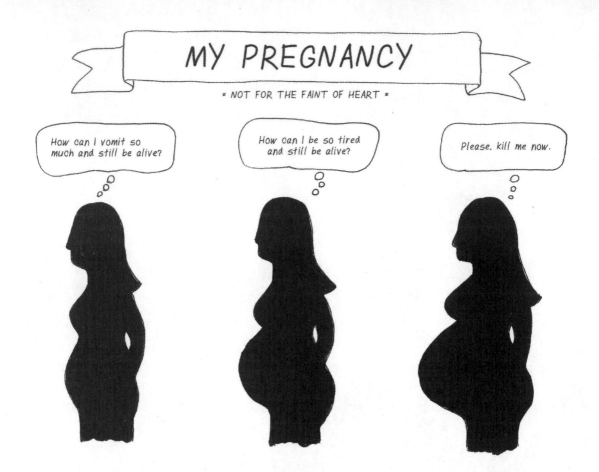

THE FIRST TRIMESTER

My most memorable bout of morning sickness—which came and went at all times of the day and night—hit just after I had drunk an entire mixed berry smoothie for breakfast at work. The vomiting was so forceful that it splashed everywhere in the bathroom stall—on the toilet seat, across the floor and all over the walls. It looked like *The Texas Chain Saw Massacre* by the time I was done.

THE SECOND TRIMESTER

I have a short torso, but you were a regular-sized fetus, which basically meant that you were living in pretty cramped quarters from the start.

I always imagined you were positioned like this in my belly:

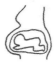

Superman style.

THE THIRD TRIMESTER

I didn't have placenta previa, but it was extremely close to blocking the cervix, so we had lots of extra ultrasounds to monitor changes as your due date got closer.

Every time I saw you on the screen, the technician would say, "She has lots of hair!"

It was thrilling to think that you were a real (hairy) person inside of me.

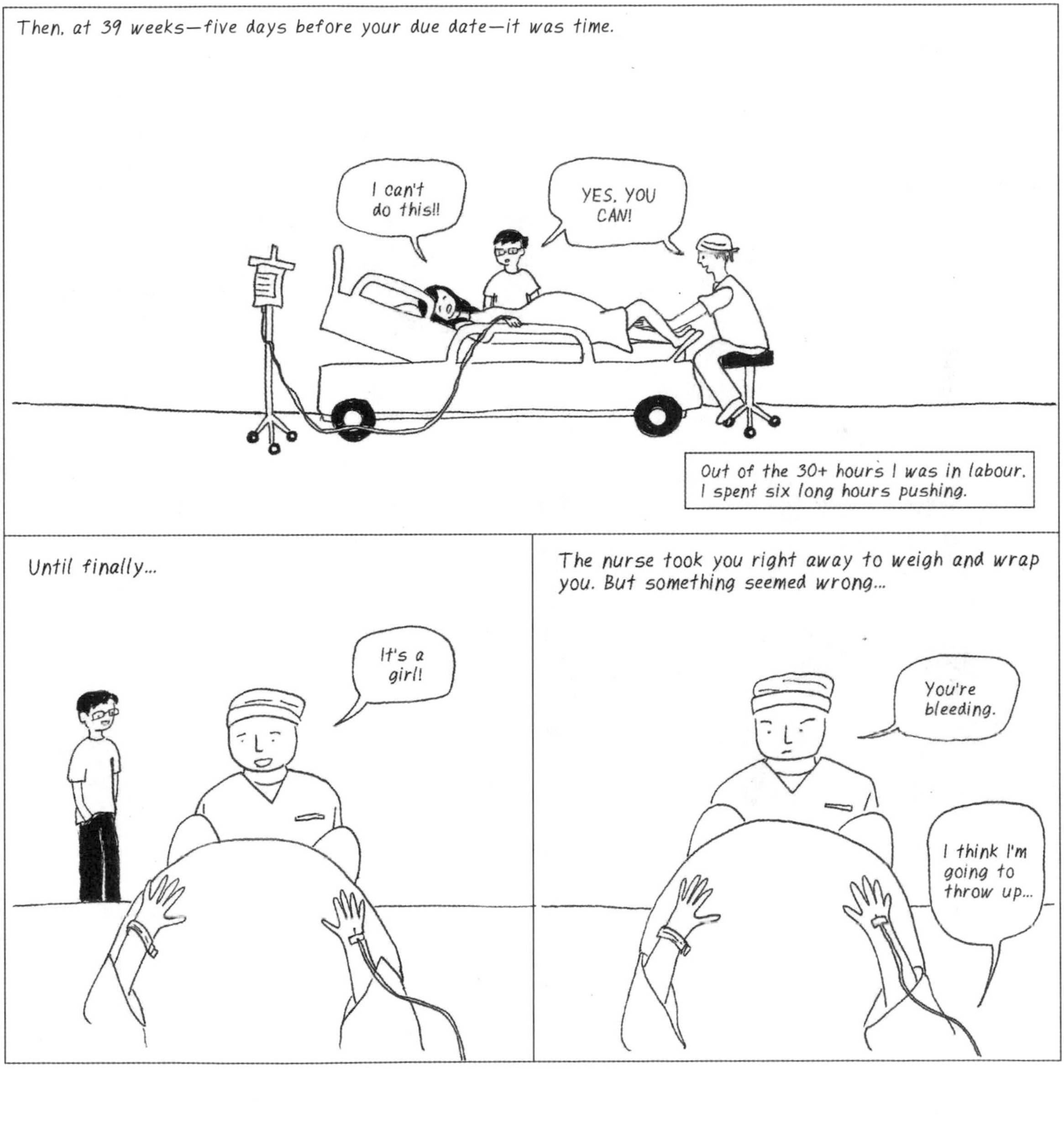
Then, at 39 weeks—five days before your due date—it was time.
I can't do this!!
YES, YOU CAN!
Out of the 30+ hours I was in labour, I spent six long hours pushing.
Until finally...
It's a girl!
The nurse took you right away to weigh and wrap you. But something seemed wrong...
You're bleeding.
I think I'm going to throw up...

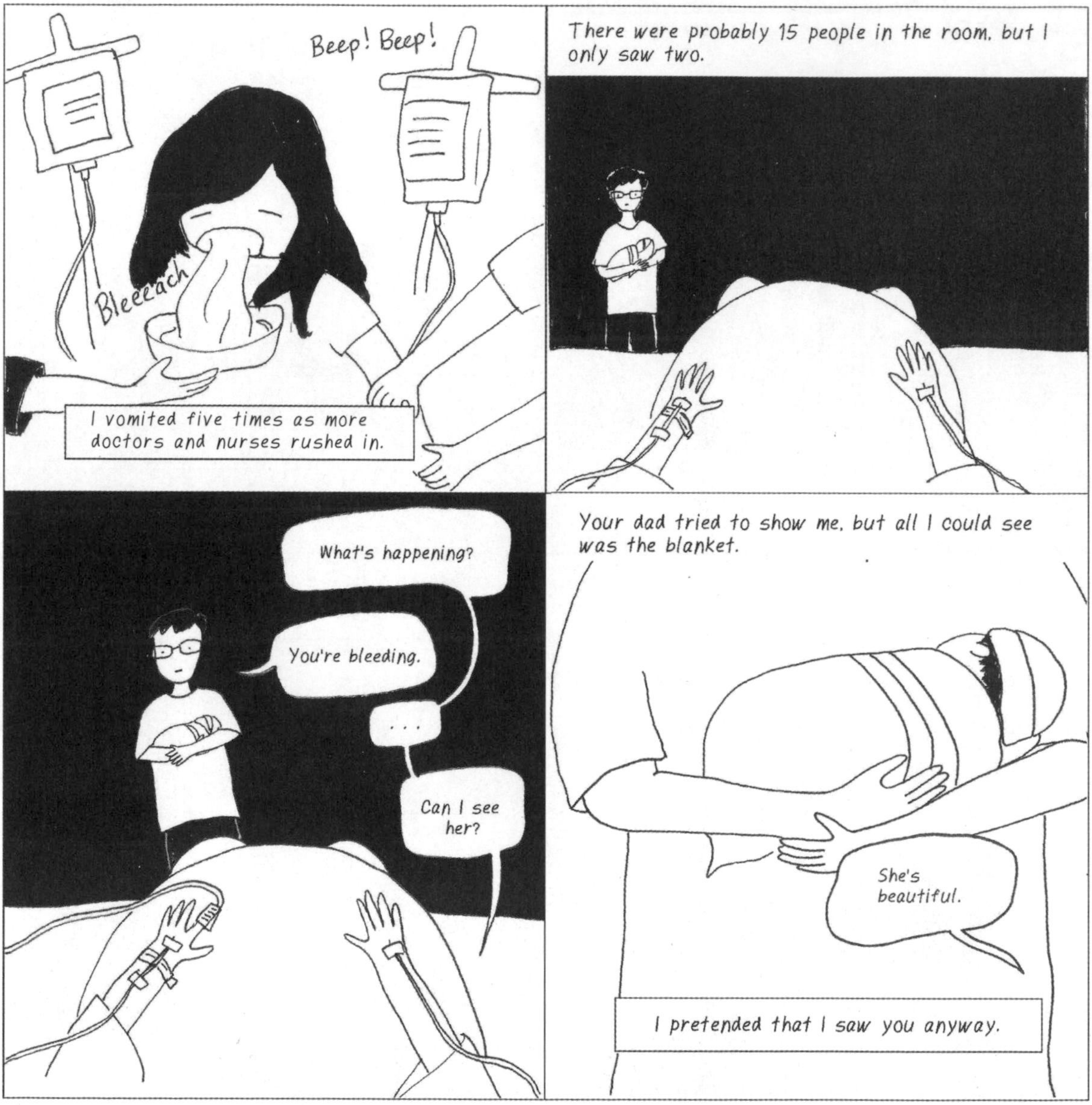
Beep! Beep!
Bleeeach
I vomited five times as more doctors and nurses rushed in.
There were probably 15 people in the room, but I only saw two.
What's happening?
You're bleeding.
. . .
Can I see her?
Your dad tried to show me, but all I could see was the blanket.
She's beautiful.
I pretended that I saw you anyway.

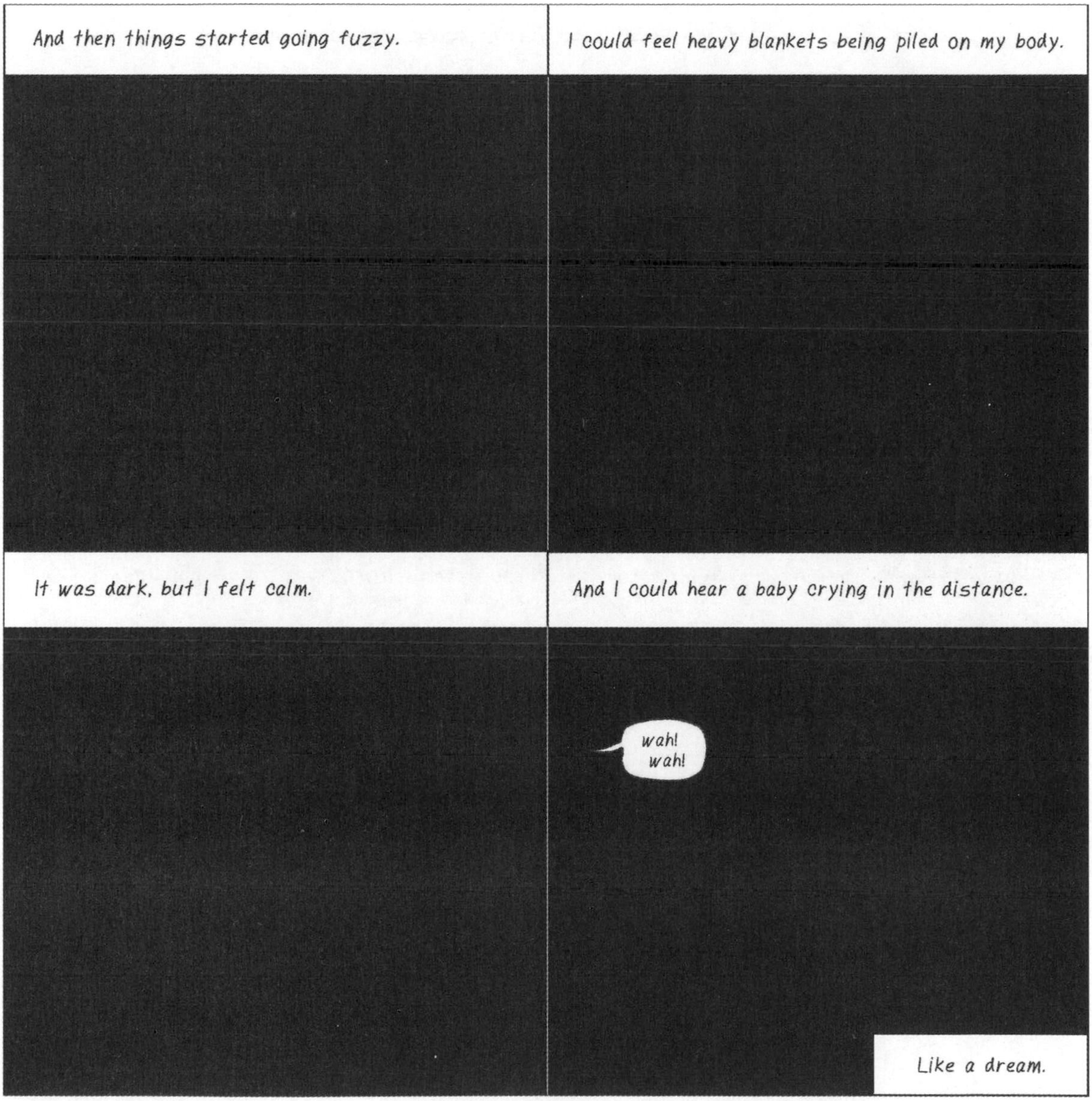
And then things started going fuzzy.
I could feel heavy blankets being piled on my body.
It was dark, but I felt calm.
And I could hear a baby crying in the distance.
wah! wah!
Like a dream.

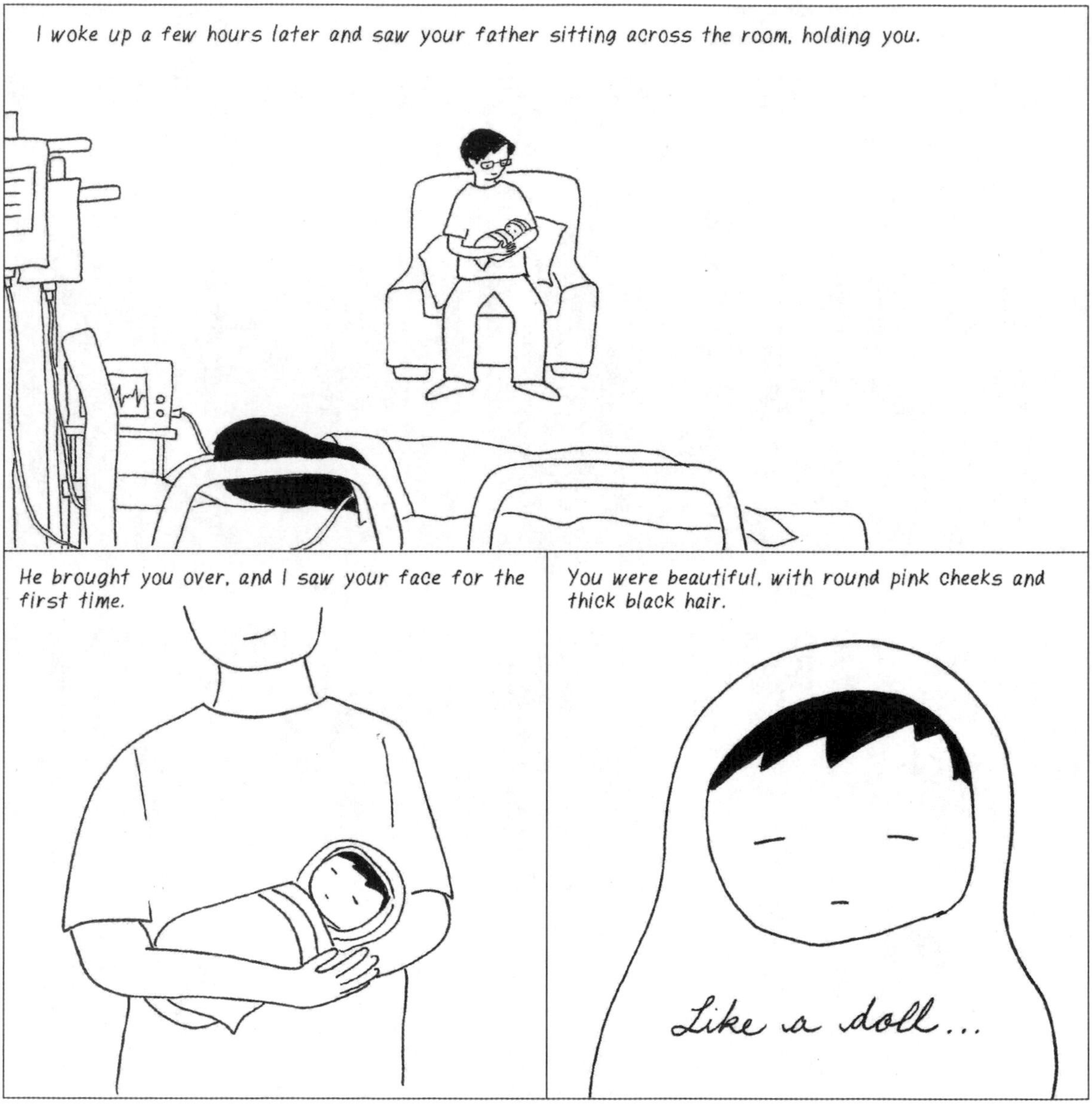
I woke up a few hours later and saw your father sitting across the room, holding you.
He brought you over, and I saw your face for the first time.
You were beautiful, with round pink cheeks and thick black hair.
Like a doll...

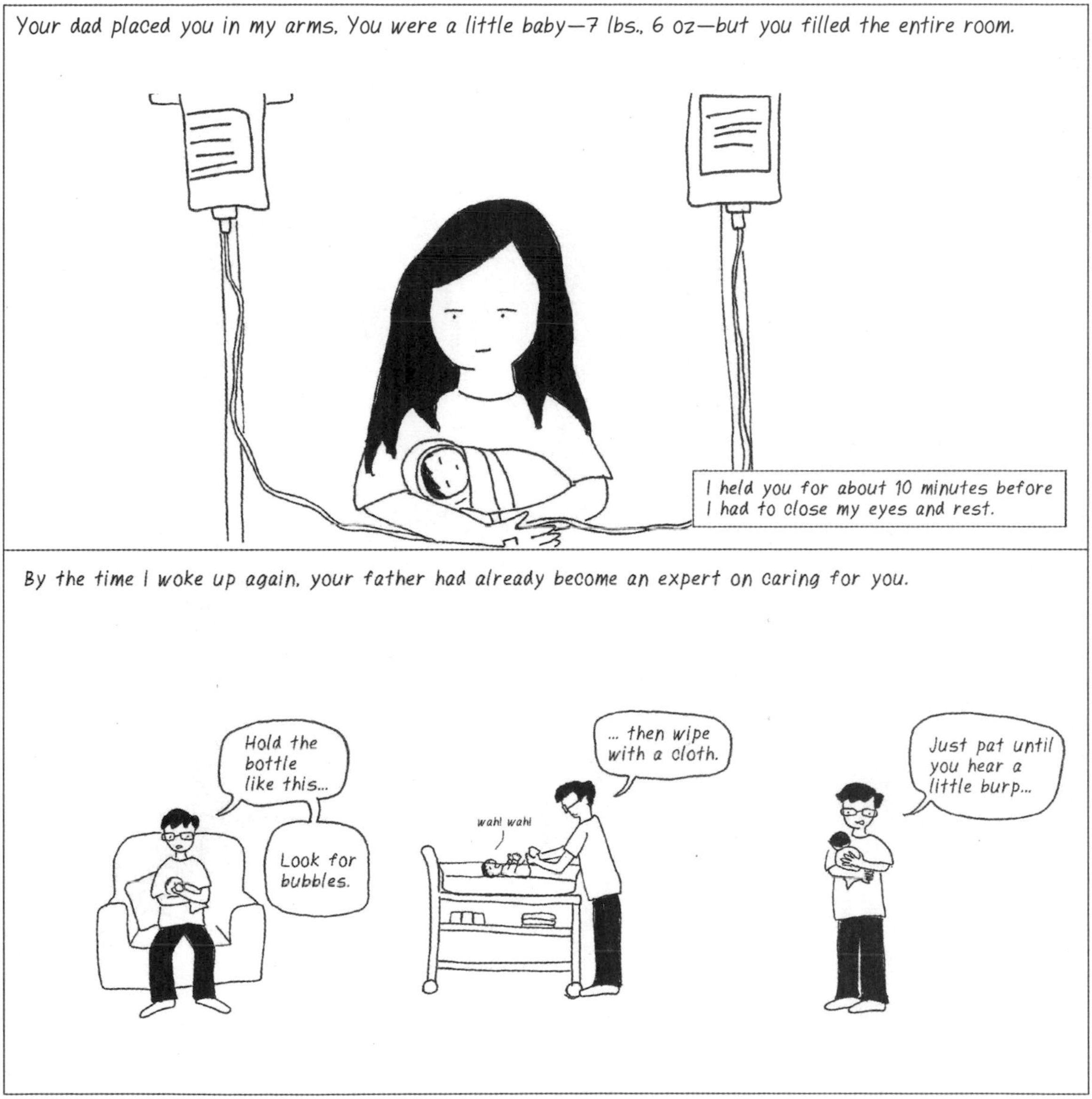
Your dad placed you in my arms. You were a little baby—7 lbs., 6 oz—but you filled the entire room.
I held you for about 10 minutes before I had to close my eyes and rest.
By the time I woke up again, your father had already become an expert on caring for you.
Hold the bottle like this...
Look for bubbles.
wah! wah!
... then wipe with a cloth.
Just pat until you hear a little burp...

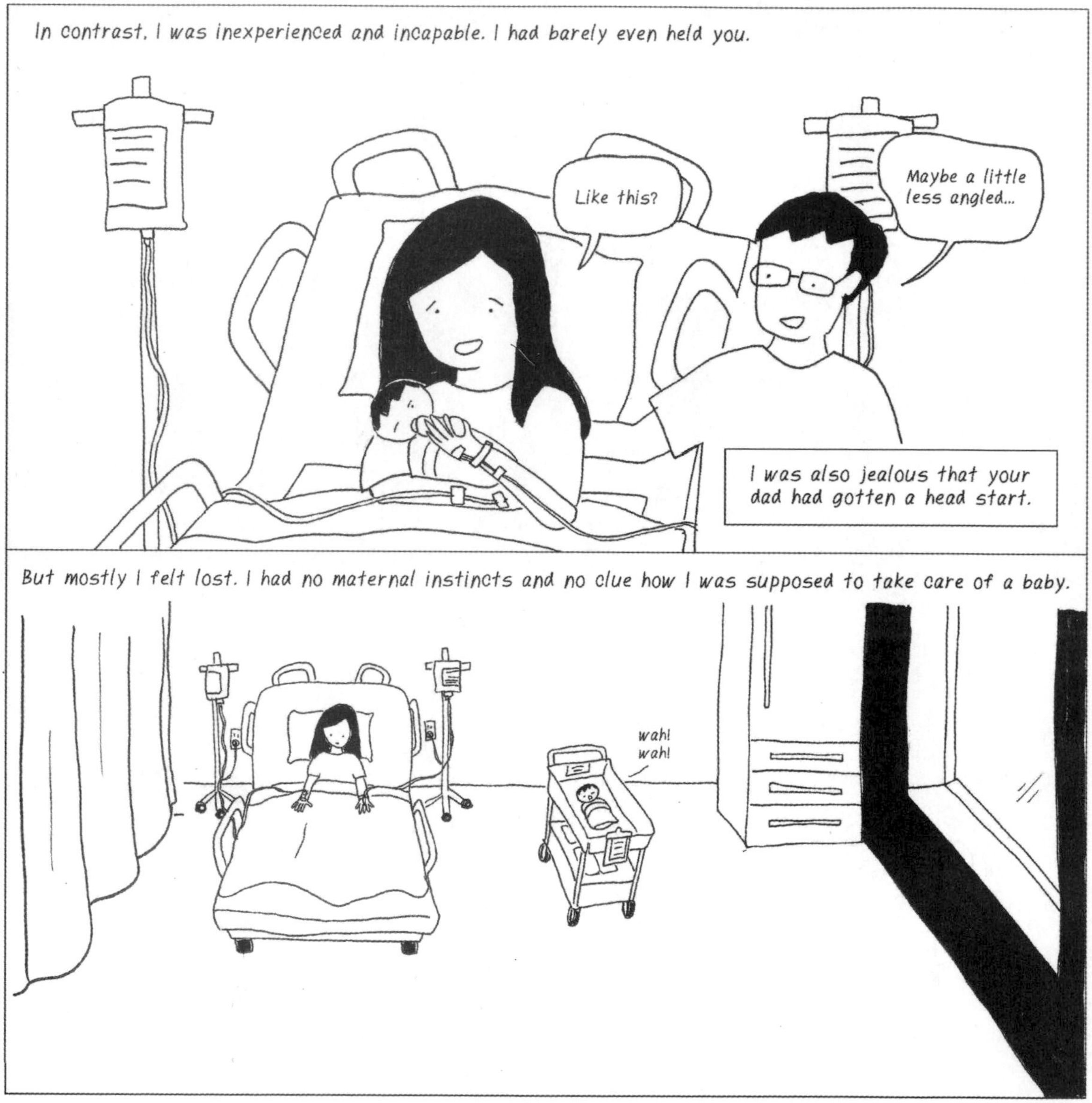
In contrast, I was inexperienced and incapable. I had barely even held you.
Like this?
Maybe a little less angled...
I was also jealous that your dad had gotten a head start.
But mostly I felt lost. I had no maternal instincts and no clue how I was supposed to take care of a baby.
wah! wah!

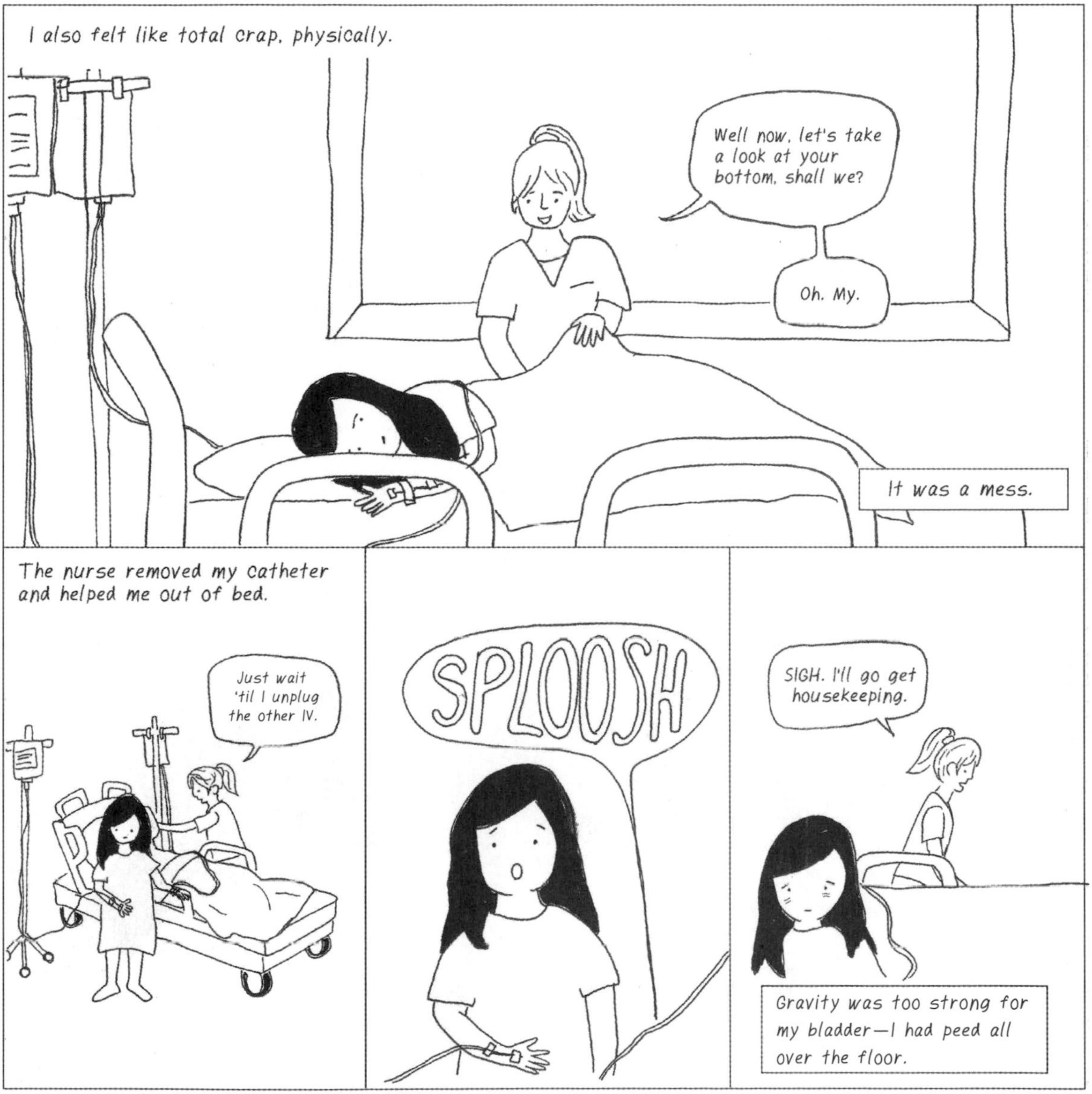
I also felt like total crap, physically.
Well now, let's take a look at your bottom, shall we?
Oh. My.
It was a mess.
The nurse removed my catheter and helped me out of bed.
Just wait 'til I unplug the other IV.
SPLOOSH
SIGH. I'll go get housekeeping.
Gravity was too strong for my bladder—I had peed all over the floor.

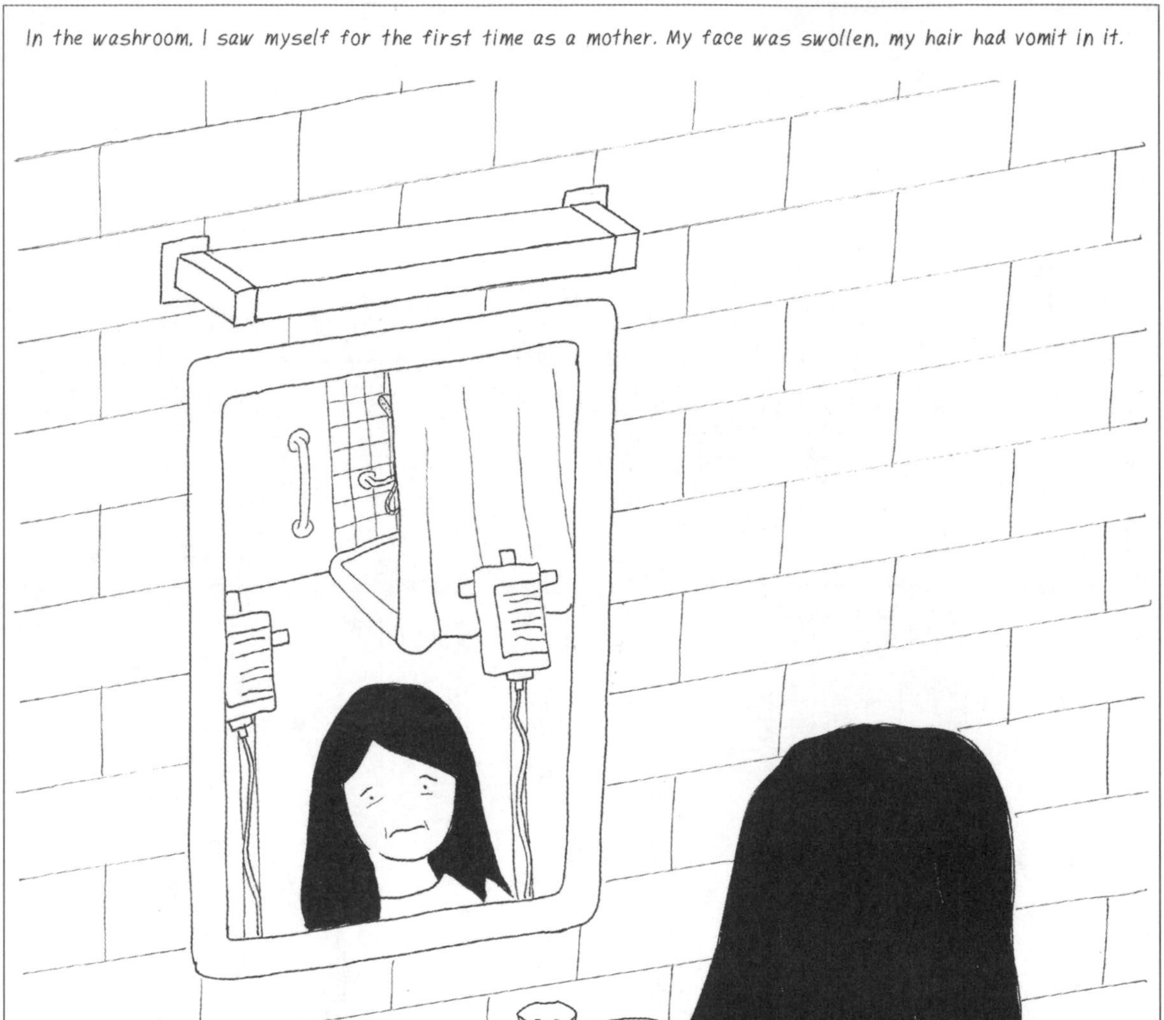
In the washroom, I saw myself for the first time as a mother. My face was swollen, my hair had vomit in it.
I looked as good as I felt.

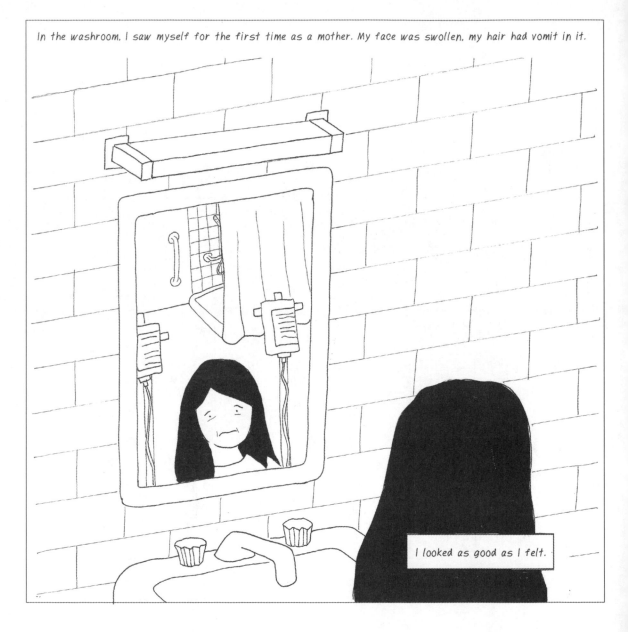

MY POSTPARTUM BODY

NOT FOR THE FAINT OF HEART

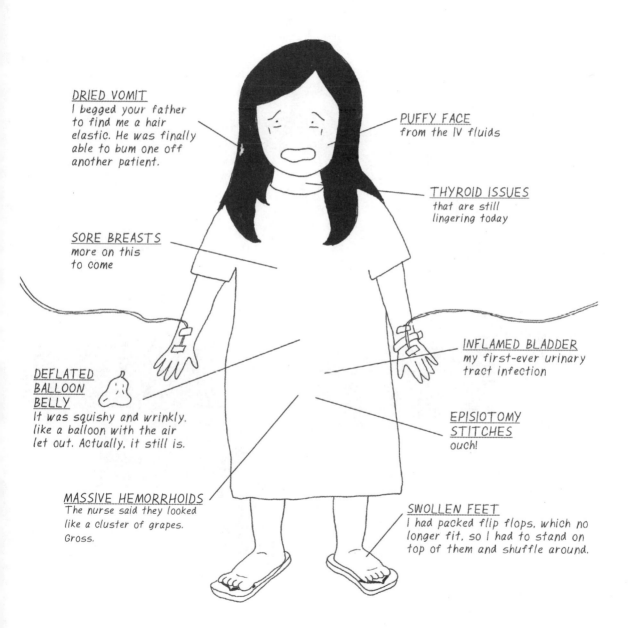

DRIED VOMIT
I begged your father to find me a hair elastic. He was finally able to bum one off another patient.

PUFFY FACE
from the IV fluids

THYROID ISSUES
that are still lingering today

SORE BREASTS
more on this to come

DEFLATED BALLOON BELLY
It was squishy and wrinkly, like a balloon with the air let out. Actually, it still is.

INFLAMED BLADDER
my first-ever urinary tract infection

EPISIOTOMY STITCHES
ouch!

MASSIVE HEMORRHOIDS
The nurse said they looked like a cluster of grapes. Gross.

SWOLLEN FEET
I had packed flip flops, which no longer fit, so I had to stand on top of them and shuffle around.

At 9 o'clock that evening, the nurse said that your father had to leave.
You'll be back first thing in the morning?
Just take her to the nursery if you need to.
I had to take care of you alone for the first time.
The minute I closed my eyes, you began to cry.
wah! wah!
I was so, so tired.

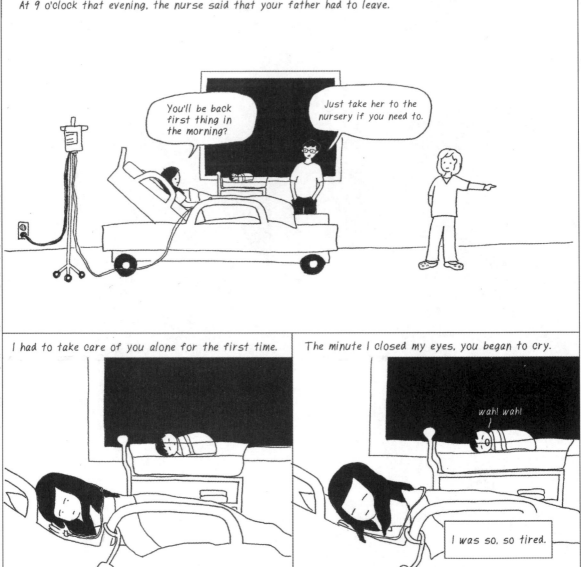

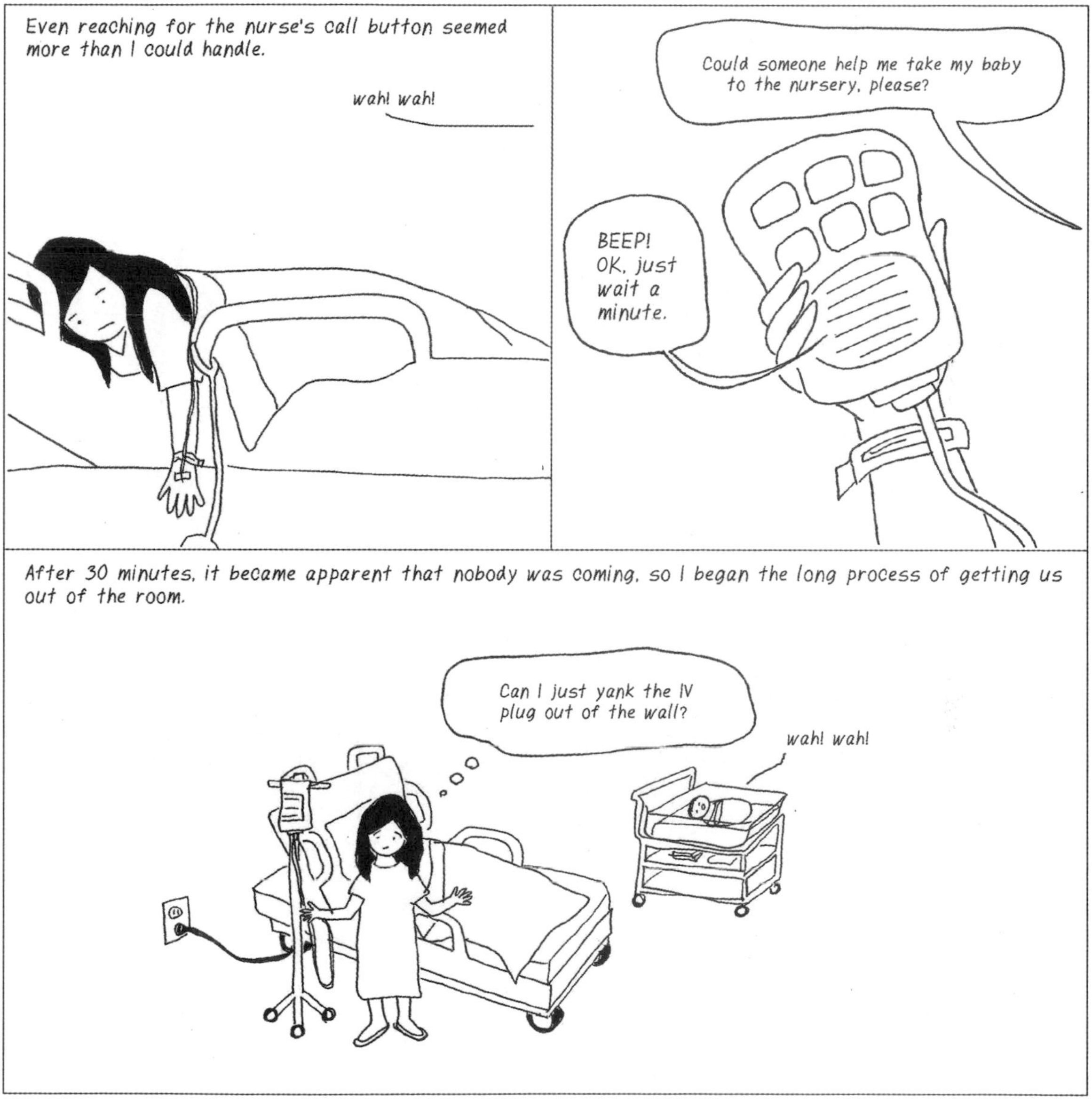
Even reaching for the nurse's call button seemed more than I could handle.
wah! wah!
Could someone help me take my baby to the nursery, please?
BEEP! OK, just wait a minute.
After 30 minutes, it became apparent that nobody was coming, so I began the long process of getting us out of the room.
Can I just yank the IV plug out of the wall?
wah! wah!

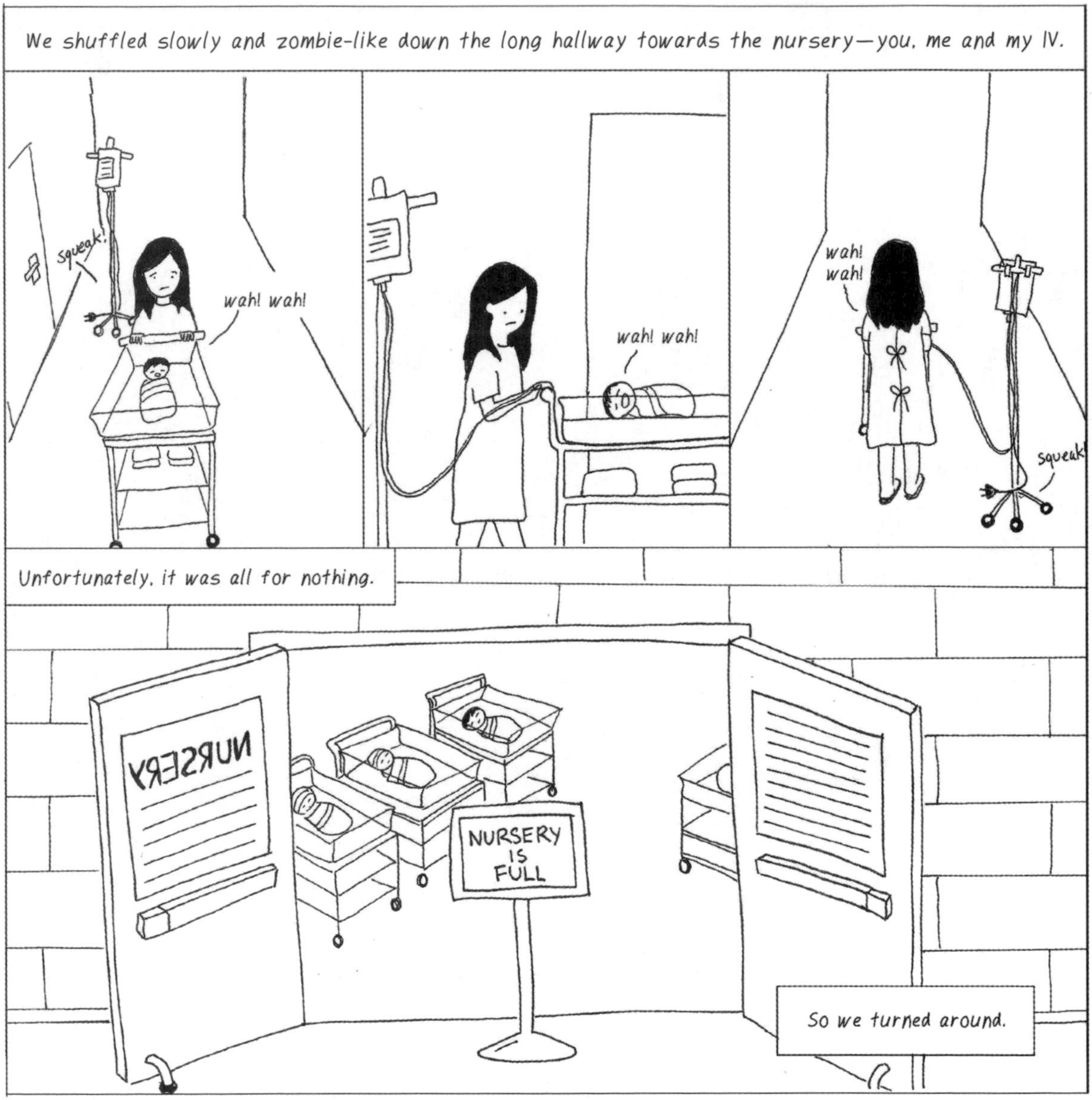
We shuffled slowly and zombie-like down the long hallway towards the nursery—you, me and my IV.
squeak!
wah! wah!
wah! wah!
wah!
wah!
squeak!
Unfortunately, it was all for nothing.
NURSERY
NURSERY IS FULL
So we turned around.

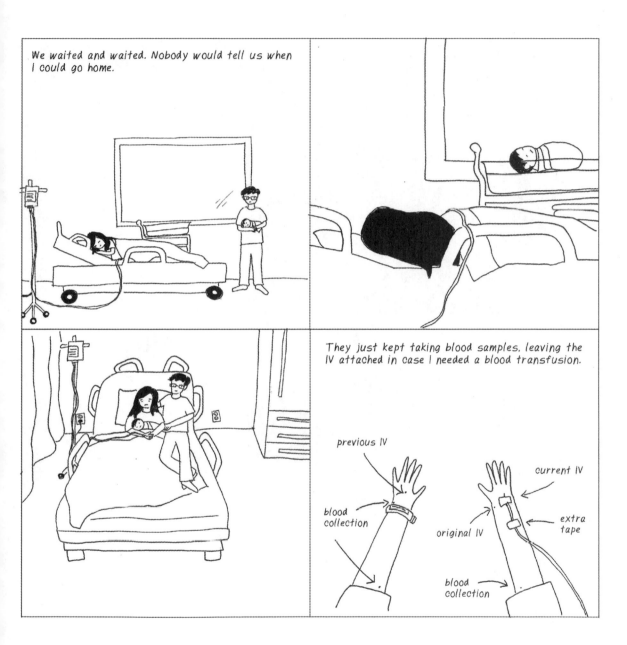

We waited and waited. Nobody would tell us when I could go home.

They just kept taking blood samples, leaving the IV attached in case I needed a blood transfusion.

previous IV

blood collection

current IV

original IV

extra tape

blood collection

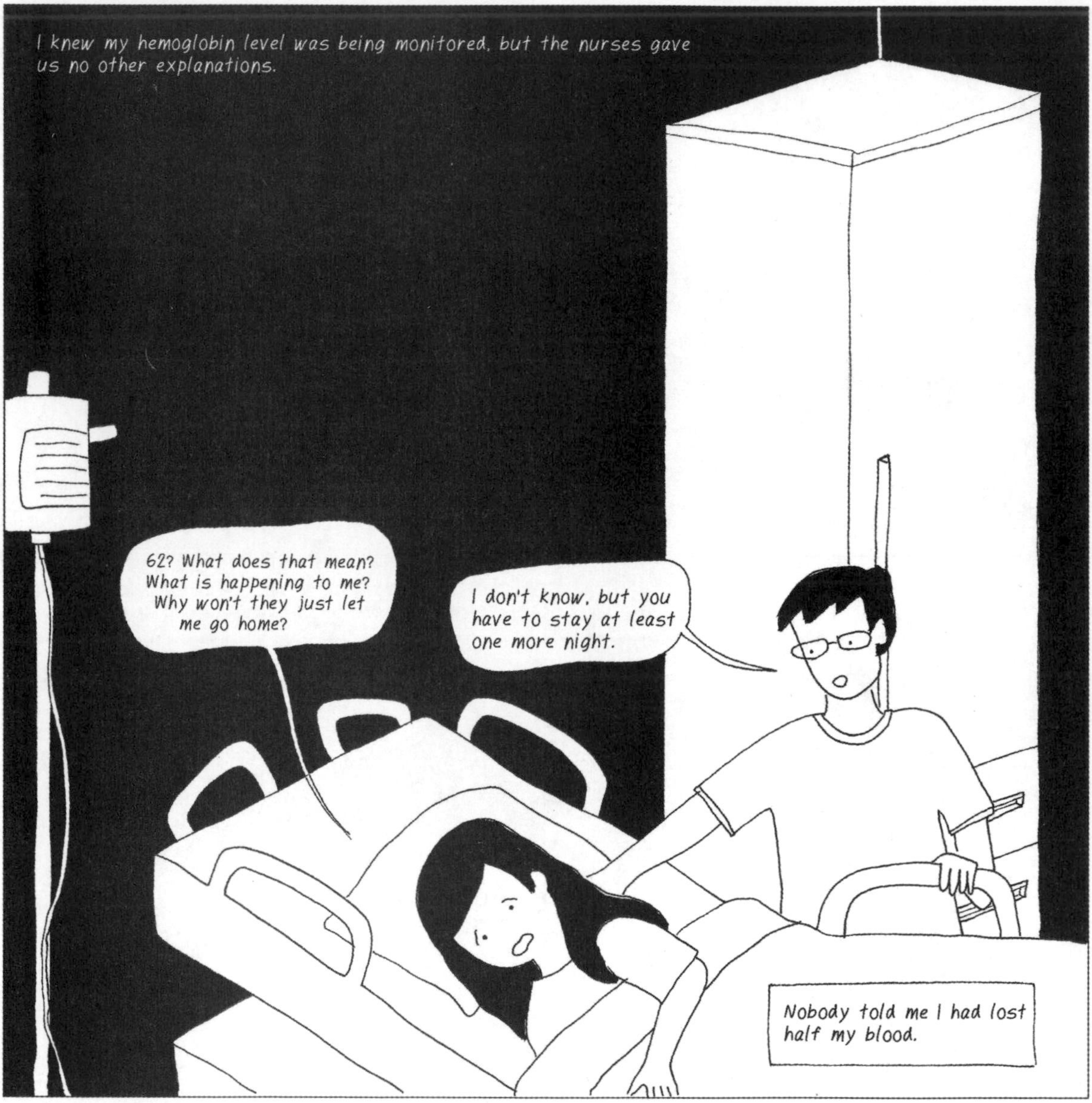
I knew my hemoglobin level was being monitored, but the nurses gave us no other explanations.
62? What does that mean? What is happening to me? Why won't they just let me go home?
I don't know, but you have to stay at least one more night.
Nobody told me I had lost half my blood.

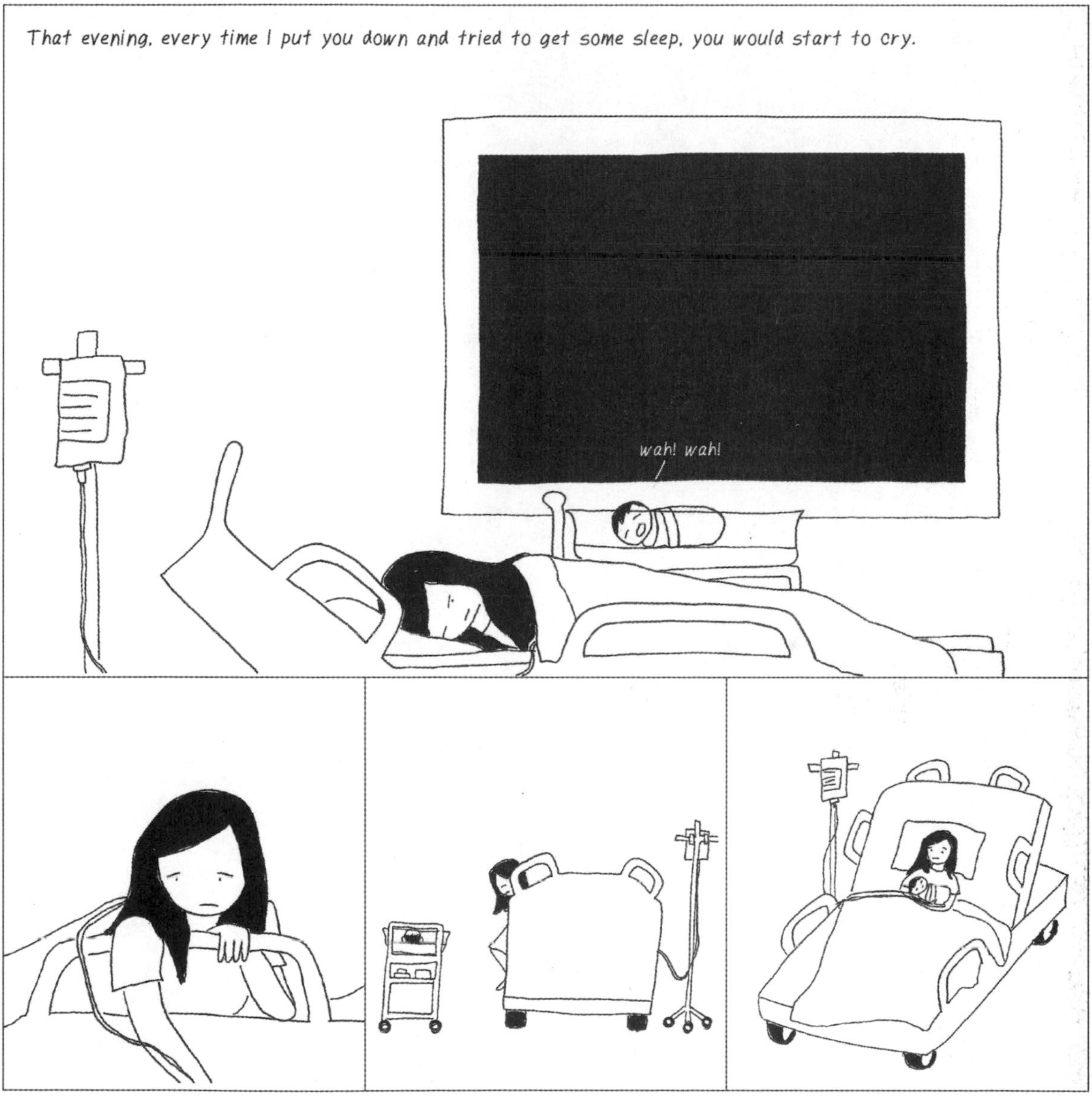
That evening, every time I put you down and tried to get some sleep, you would start to cry.
wah! wah!

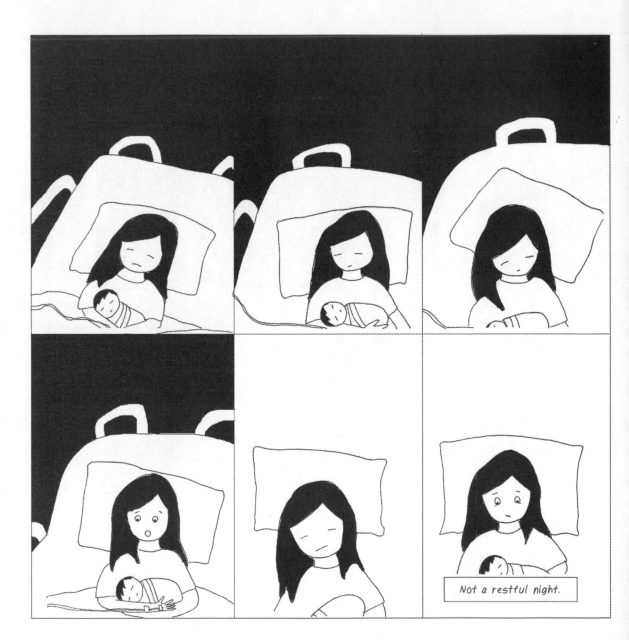

Not a restful night.

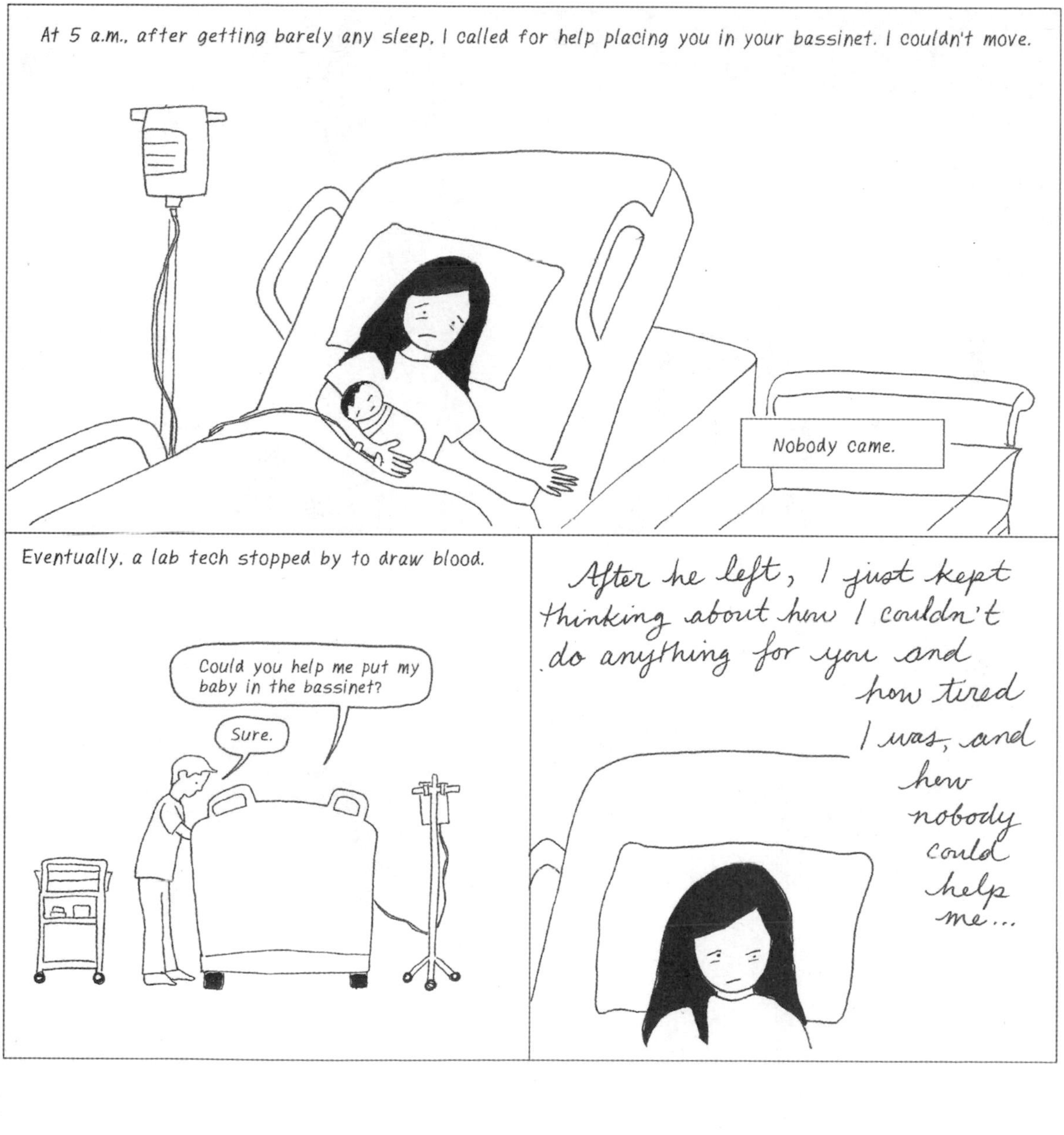
At 5 a.m., after getting barely any sleep, I called for help placing you in your bassinet. I couldn't move.
Nobody came.
Eventually, a lab tech stopped by to draw blood.
Could you help me put my baby in the bassinet?
Sure.
After he left, I just kept thinking about how I couldn't do anything for you and how tired I was, and how nobody could help me...

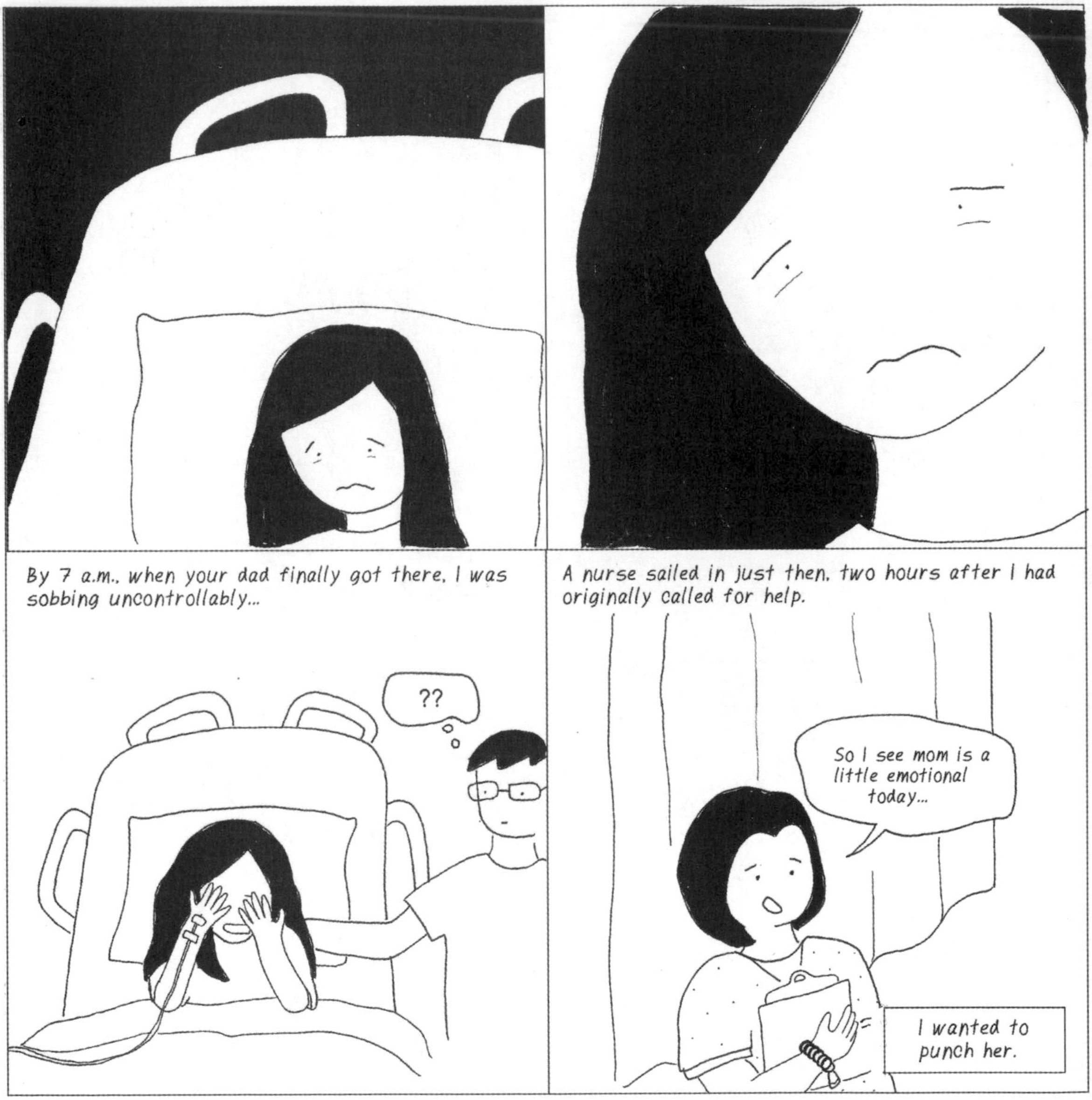
By 7 a.m., when your dad finally got there, I was sobbing uncontrollably...
??
A nurse sailed in just then, two hours after I had originally called for help.
So I see mom is a little emotional today...
I wanted to punch her.

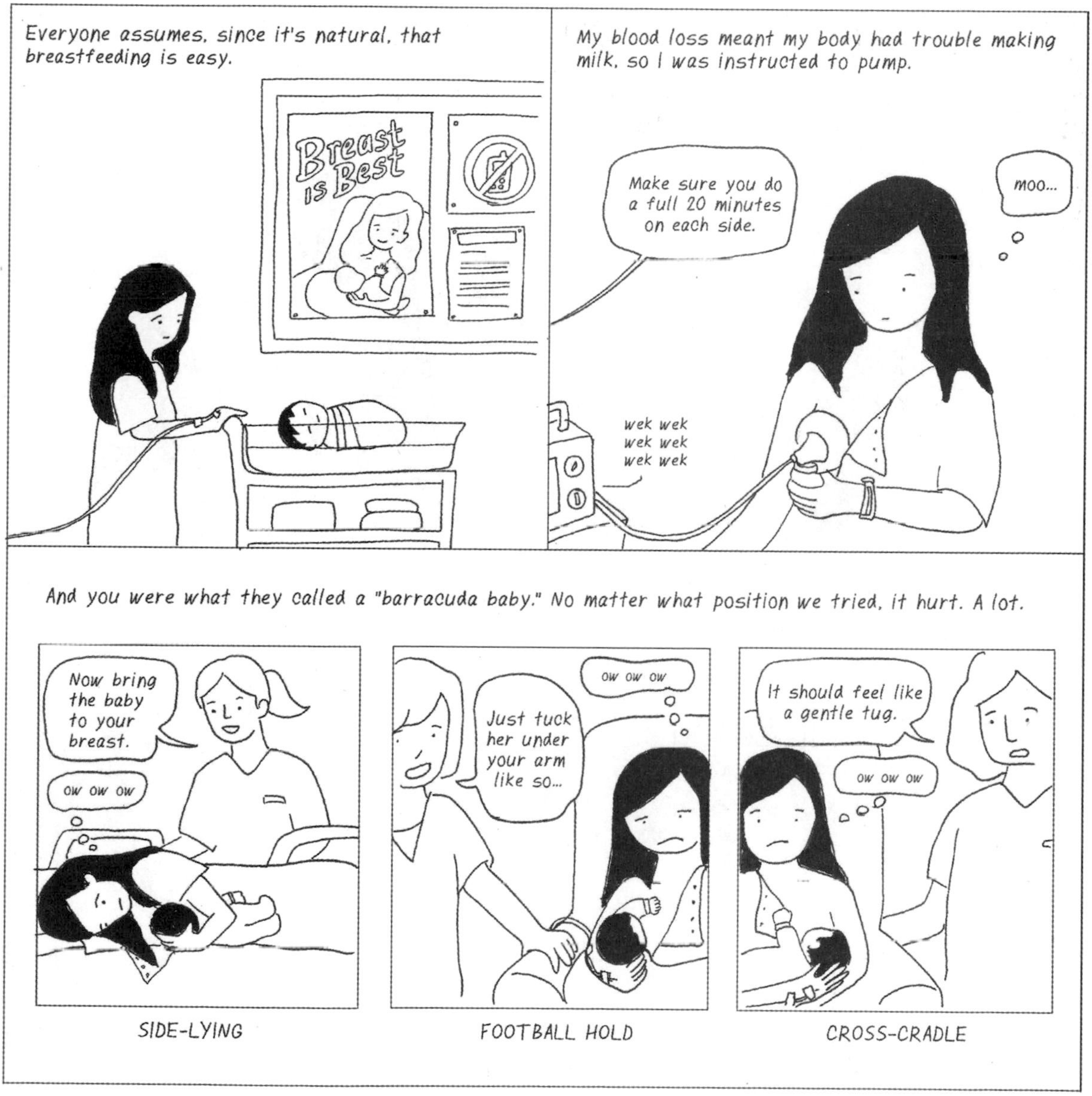
Everyone assumes, since it's natural, that breastfeeding is easy.
Breast is Best
My blood loss meant my body had trouble making milk, so I was instructed to pump.
Make sure you do a full 20 minutes on each side.
moo...
wek wek
wek wek
wek wek
And you were what they called a "barracuda baby." No matter what position we tried, it hurt. A lot.
Now bring the baby to your breast.
ow ow ow
SIDE-LYING
Just tuck her under your arm like so...
ow ow ow
FOOTBALL HOLD
It should feel like a gentle tug.
ow ow ow
CROSS-CRADLE

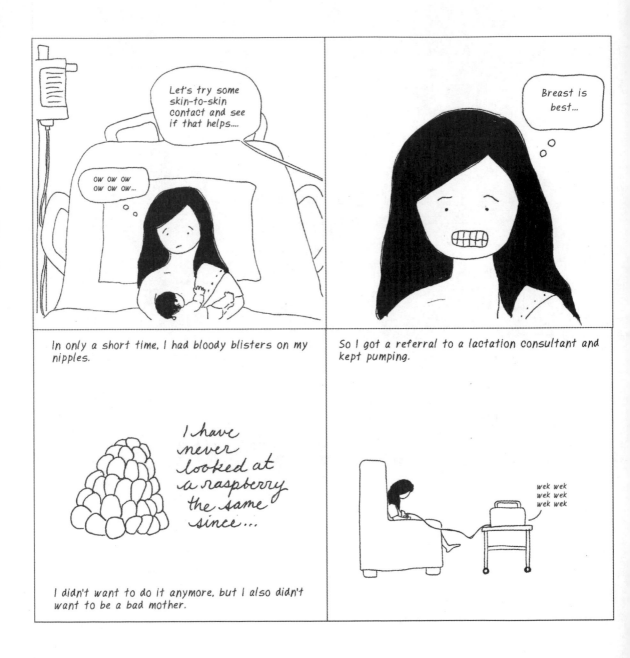

Let's try some skin-to-skin contact and see if that helps....
ow ow ow ow ow ow...
Breast is best...
In only a short time, I had bloody blisters on my nipples.
I have never looked at a raspberry the same since...
I didn't want to do it anymore, but I also didn't want to be a bad mother.
So I got a referral to a lactation consultant and kept pumping.
wek wek wek wek wek wek

We left the hospital when you were three days old.
MUST BUY BOTTLES & FORMULA
CAN'T BELIEVE THEY FINALLY LET US GO
EEP
HOW WILL WE KEEP HER ALIVE
I HOPE WE'RE READY
GET IRON PILLS & STOOL SOFTENER
EEP

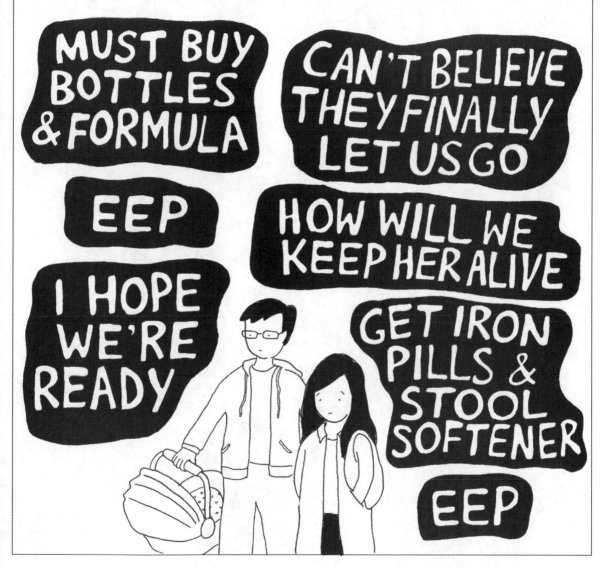

OK, you two wait here while I bring the car around.

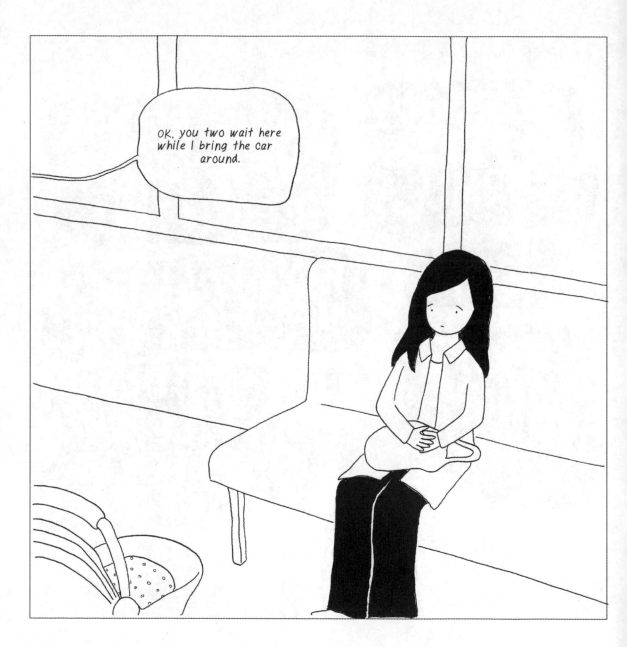

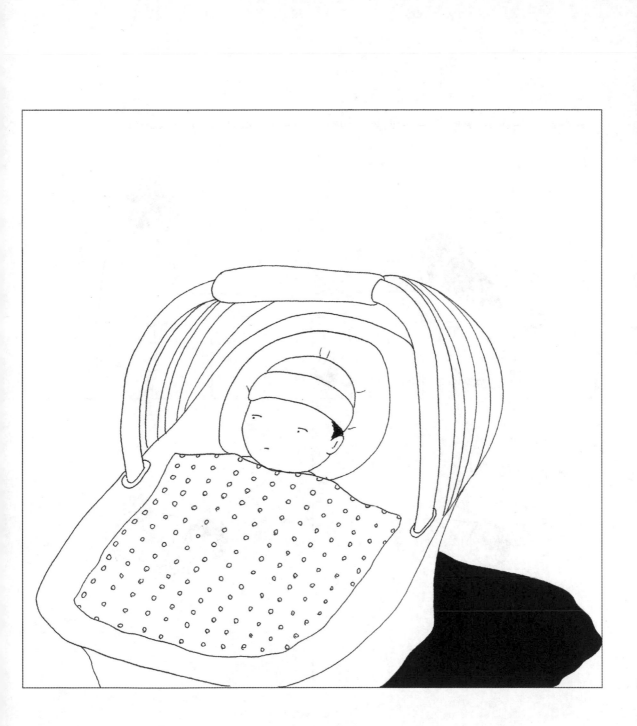

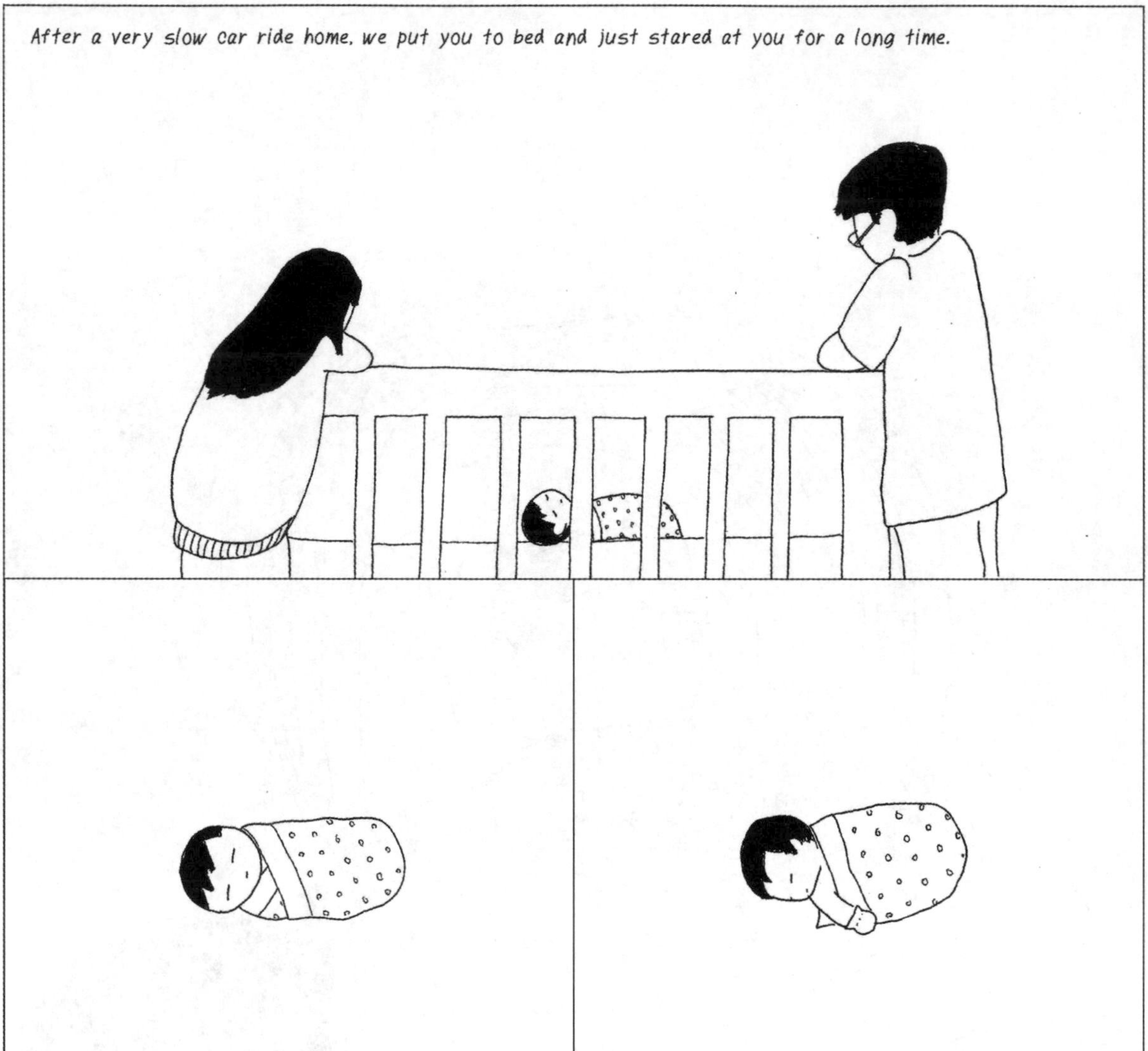
After a very slow car ride home, we put you to bed and just stared at you for a long time.

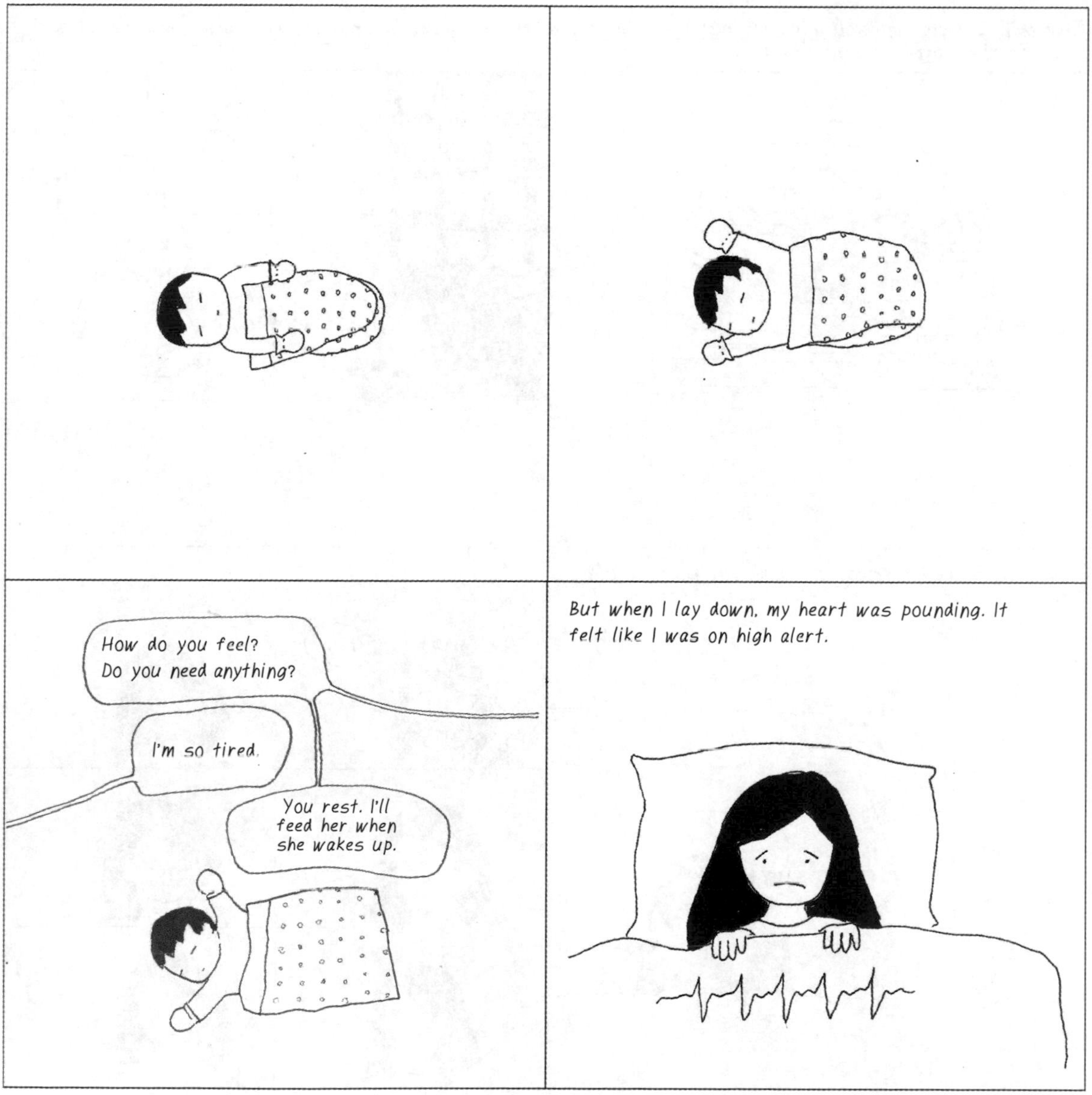
How do you feel?
Do you need anything?
I'm so tired.
You rest. I'll feed her when she wakes up.
But when I lay down, my heart was pounding. It felt like I was on high alert.

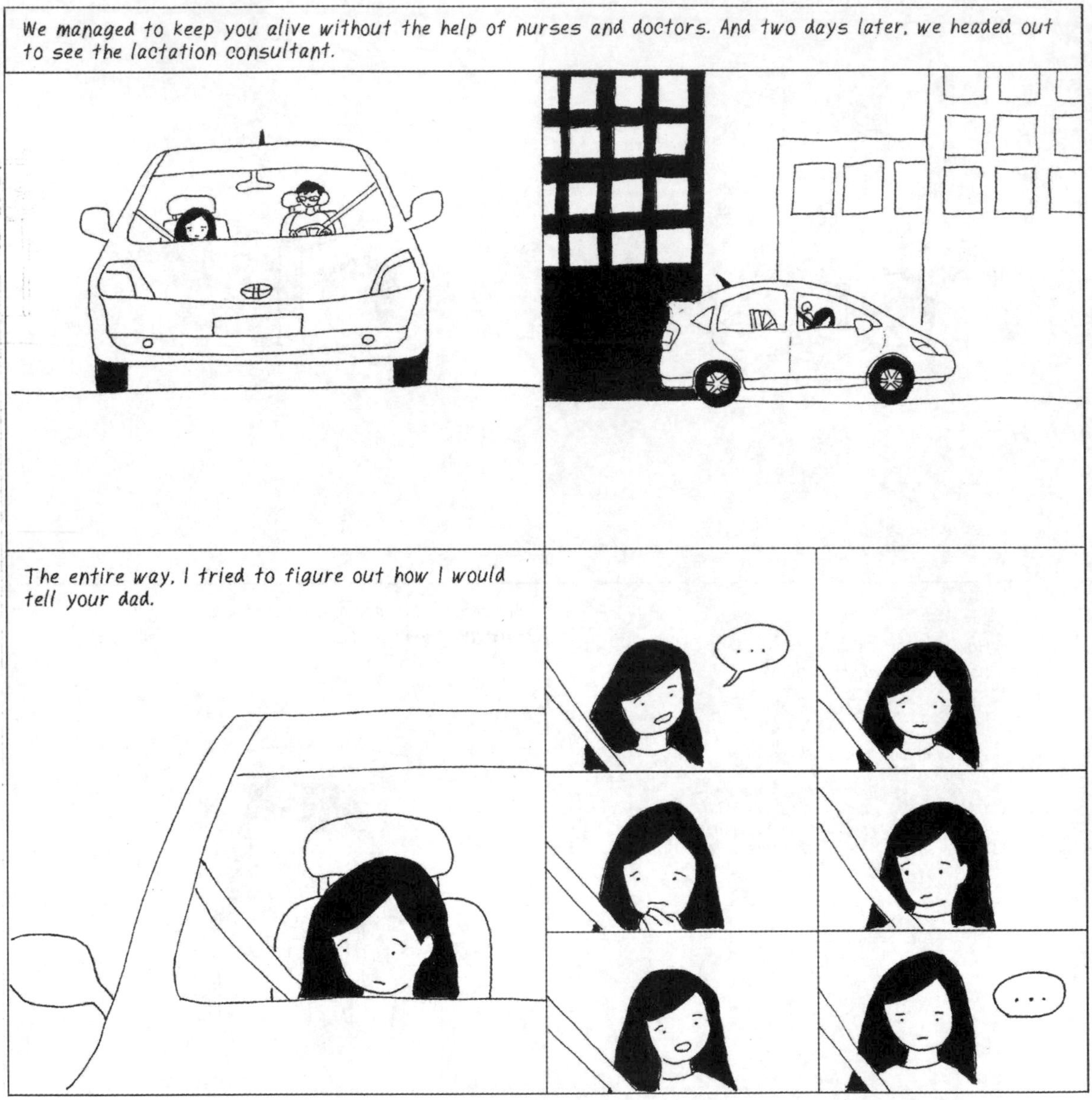
We managed to keep you alive without the help of nurses and doctors. And two days later, we headed out to see the lactation consultant.
The entire way, I tried to figure out how I would tell your dad.
...
...

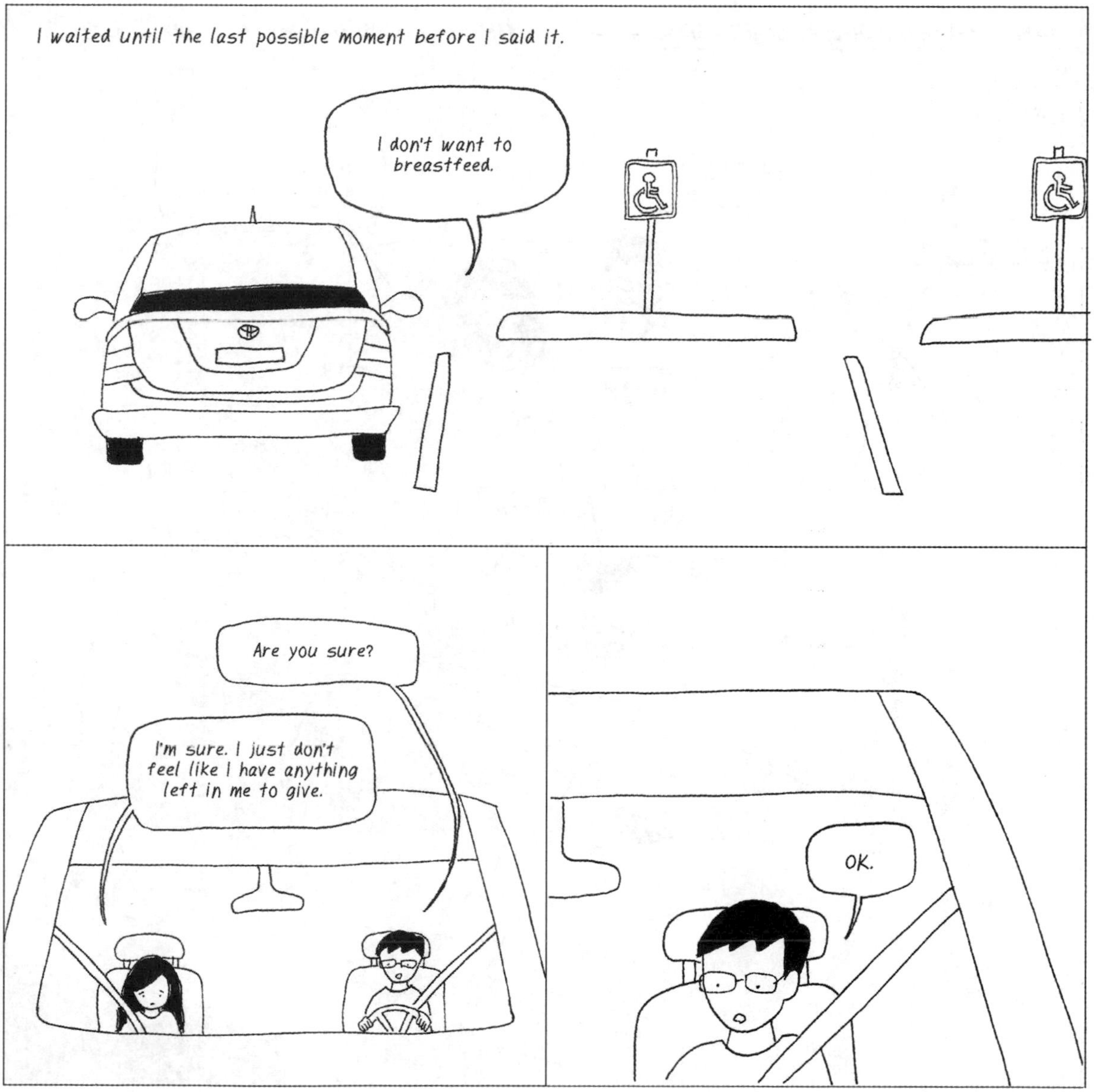
I waited until the last possible moment before I said it.
I don't want to breastfeed.
Are you sure?
I'm sure. I just don't feel like I have anything left in me to give.
OK.

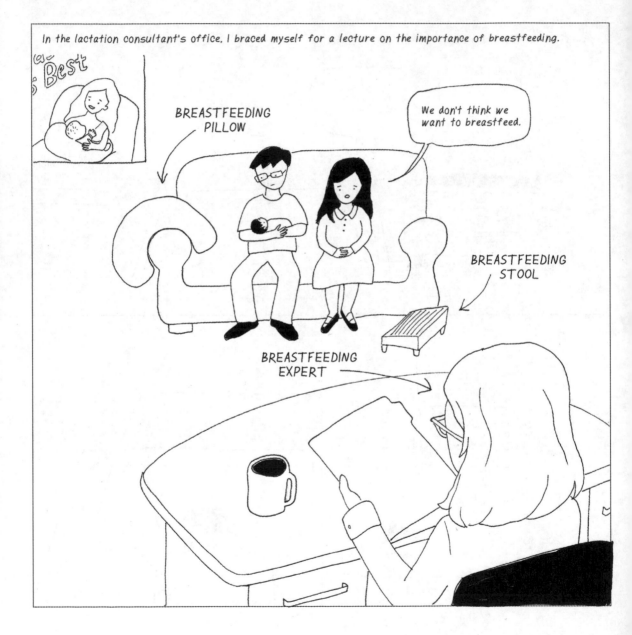

In the lactation consultant's office, I braced myself for a lecture on the importance of breastfeeding.
Best
BREASTFEEDING PILLOW
We don't think we want to breastfeed.
BREASTFEEDING STOOL
BREASTFEEDING EXPERT

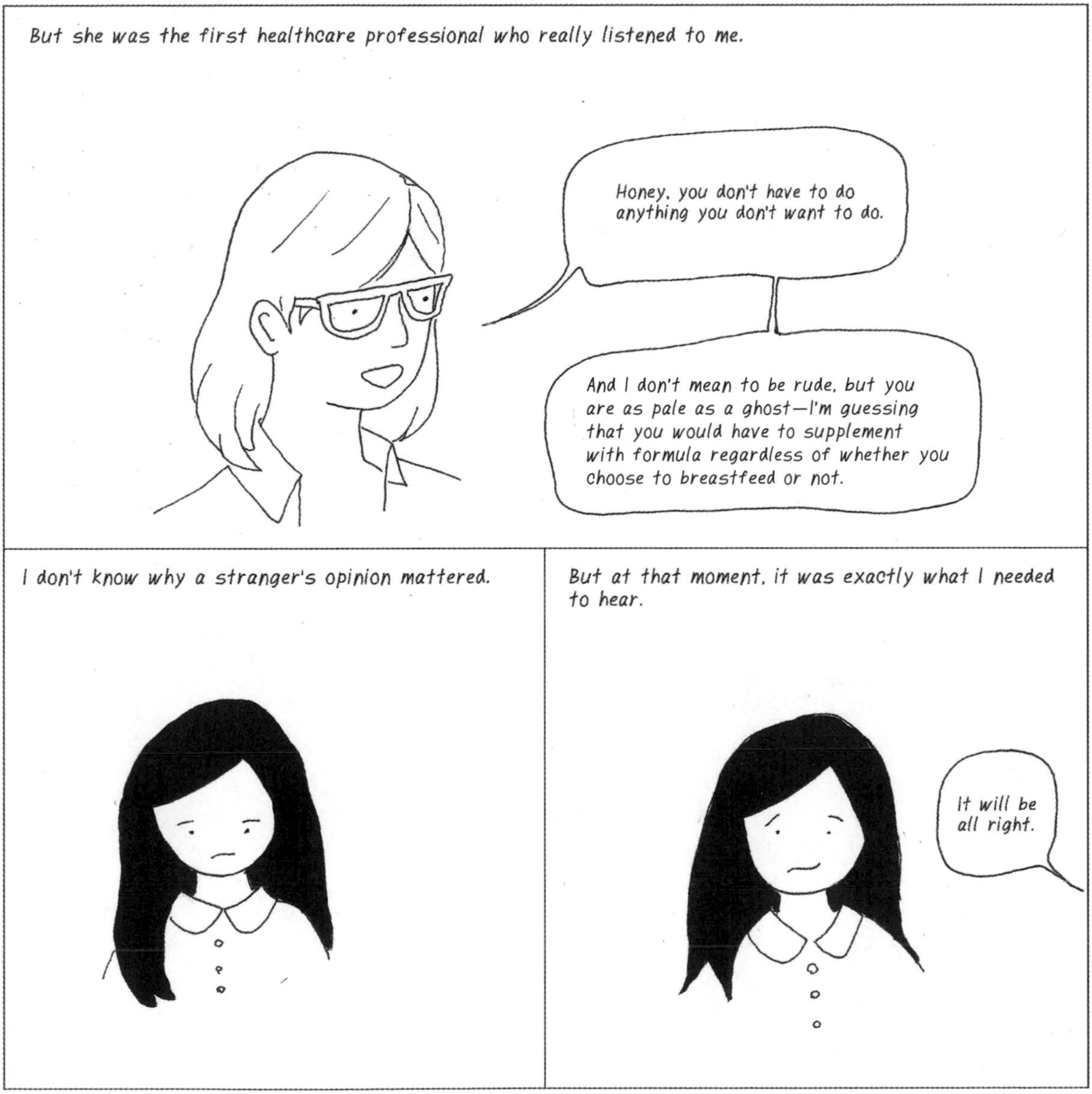
But she was the first healthcare professional who really listened to me.
Honey, you don't have to do anything you don't want to do.
And I don't mean to be rude, but you are as pale as a ghost—I'm guessing that you would have to supplement with formula regardless of whether you choose to breastfeed or not.
I don't know why a stranger's opinion mattered.
But at that moment, it was exactly what I needed to hear.
It will be all right.

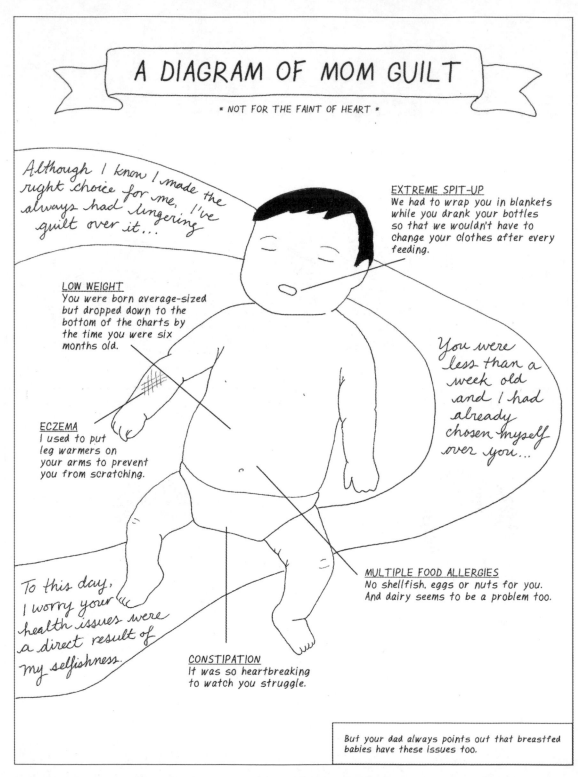

A DIAGRAM OF MOM GUILT

* NOT FOR THE FAINT OF HEART *

Although I know I made the right choice for me, I've always had lingering guilt over it...

EXTREME SPIT-UP
We had to wrap you in blankets while you drank your bottles so that we wouldn't have to change your clothes after every feeding.

LOW WEIGHT
You were born average-sized but dropped down to the bottom of the charts by the time you were six months old.

You were less than a week old and I had already chosen myself over you...

ECZEMA
I used to put leg warmers on your arms to prevent you from scratching.

MULTIPLE FOOD ALLERGIES
No shellfish, eggs or nuts for you. And dairy seems to be a problem too.

To this day, I worry your health issues were a direct result of my selfishness.

CONSTIPATION
It was so heartbreaking to watch you struggle.

But your dad always points out that breastfed babies have these issues too.

The decision took its toll on my own body as well. My milk eventually came in fully, and suddenly....

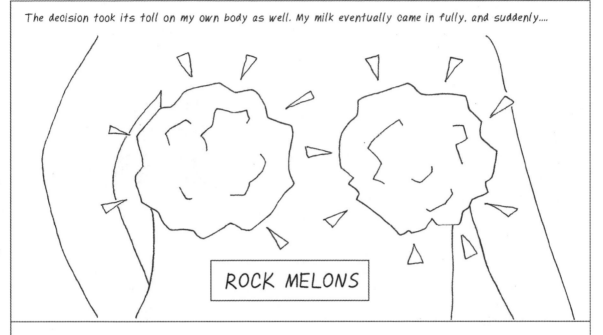

ROCK MELONS

If a baby isn't emptying your breasts, they become painfully engorged. Things that supposedly help include:

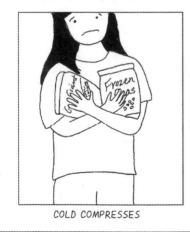

COLD COMPRESSES

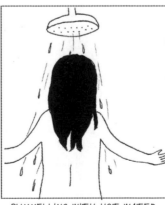

PUMMELLING WITH HOT WATER

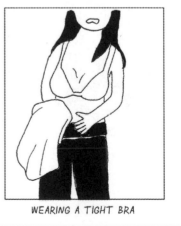

WEARING A TIGHT BRA

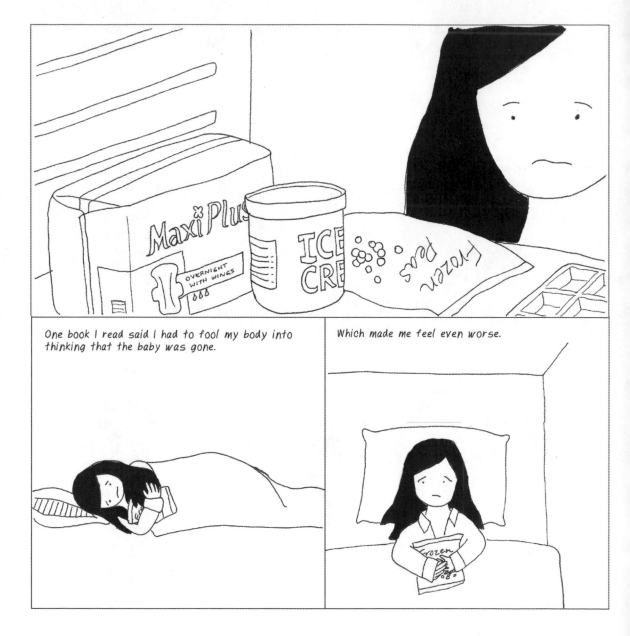

Maxi Plus
OVERNIGHT WITH WINGS
ICE CRE
Frozen peas
One book I read said I had to fool my body into thinking that the baby was gone.
Which made me feel even worse.
Frozen

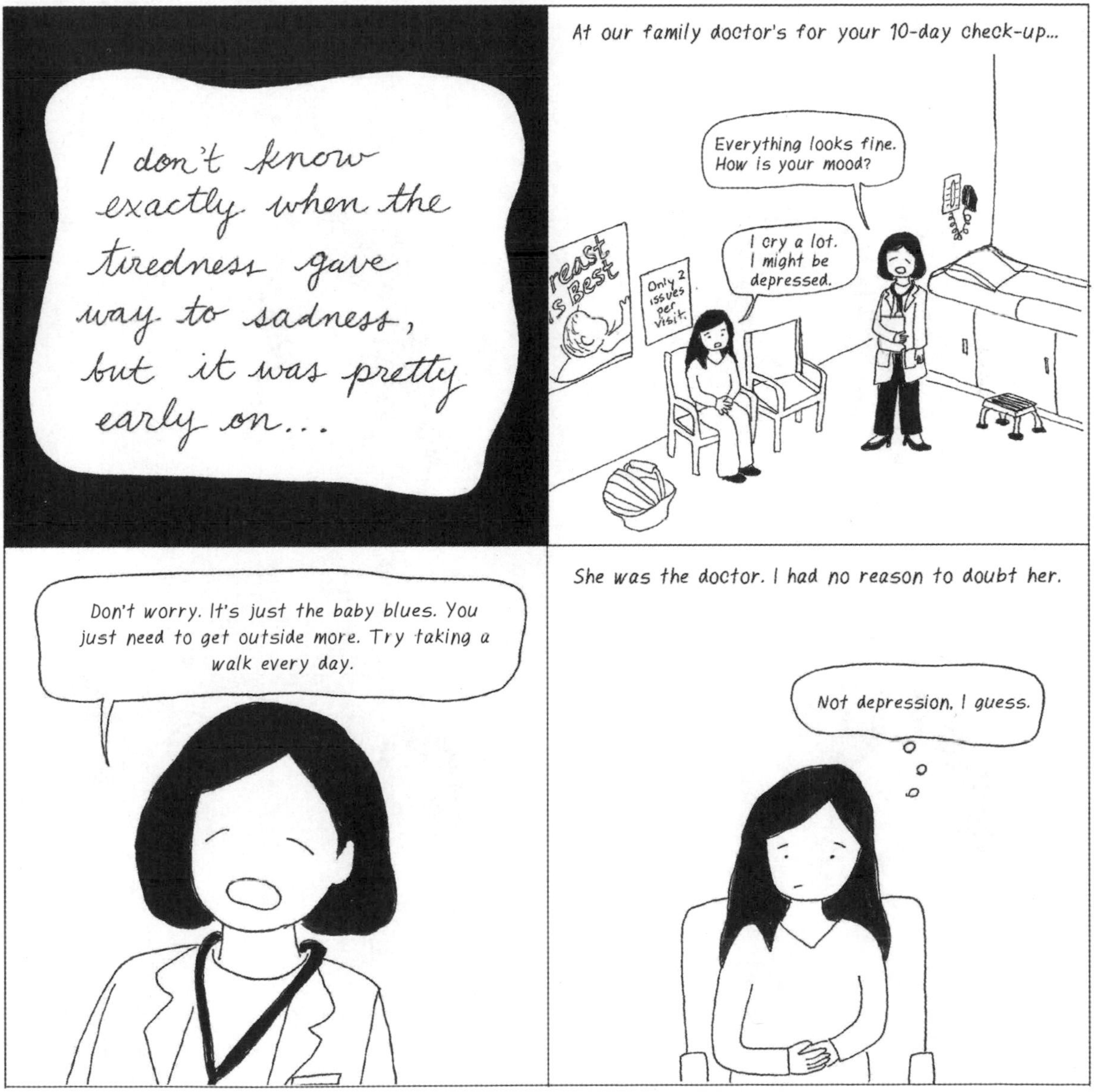
I don't know exactly when the tiredness gave way to sadness, but it was pretty early on...
At our family doctor's for your 10-day check-up...
Everything looks fine. How is your mood?
I cry a lot. I might be depressed.
Only 2 issues per visit.
Don't worry. It's just the baby blues. You just need to get outside more. Try taking a walk every day.
She was the doctor. I had no reason to doubt her.
Not depression, I guess.

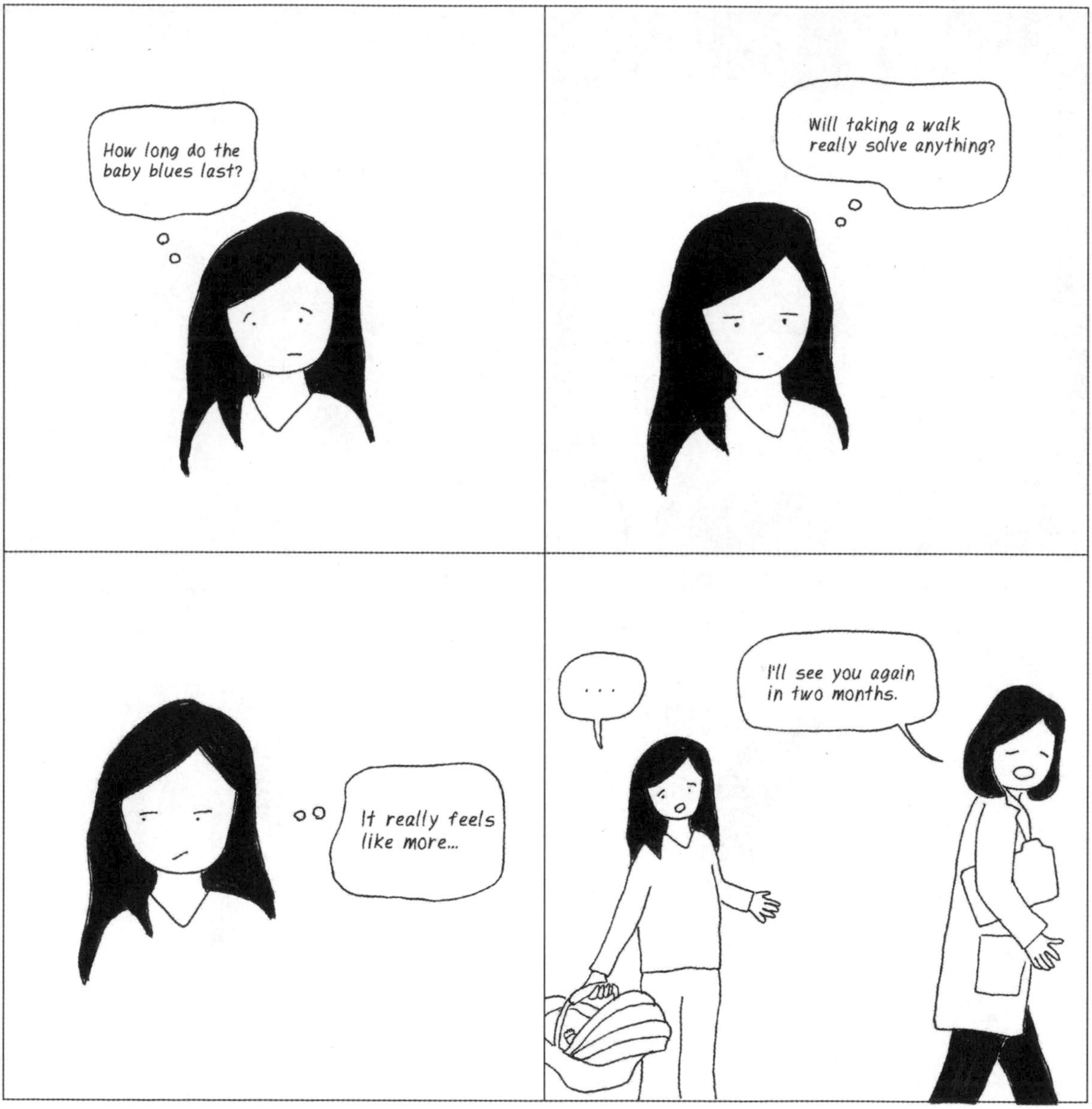

How long do the baby blues last?
Will taking a walk really solve anything?
It really feels like more...
. . .
I'll see you again in two months.

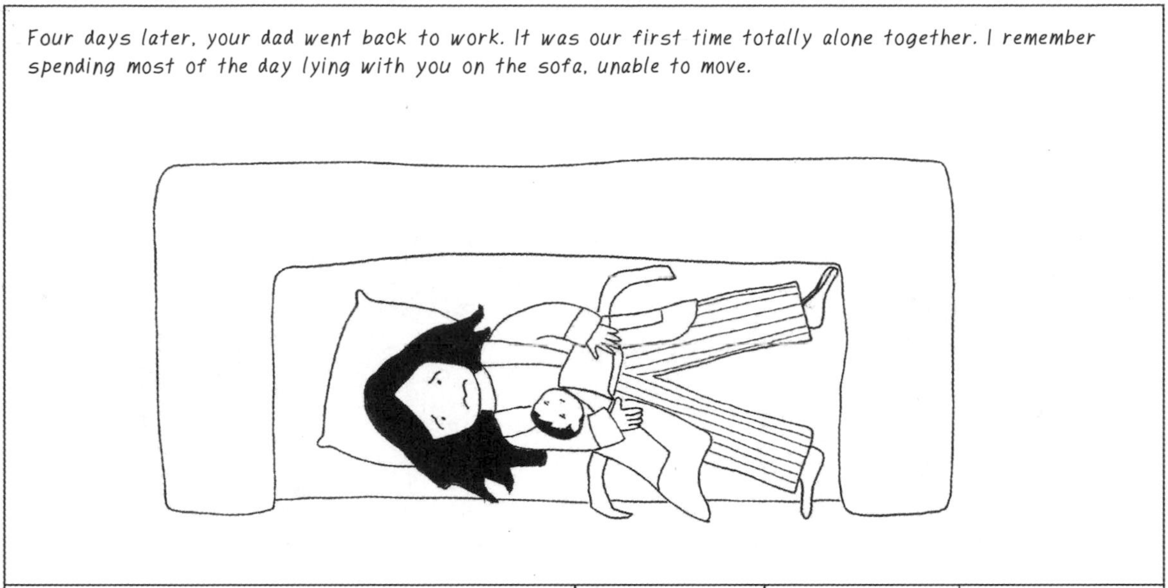
Four days later, your dad went back to work. It was our first time totally alone together. I remember spending most of the day lying with you on the sofa, unable to move.

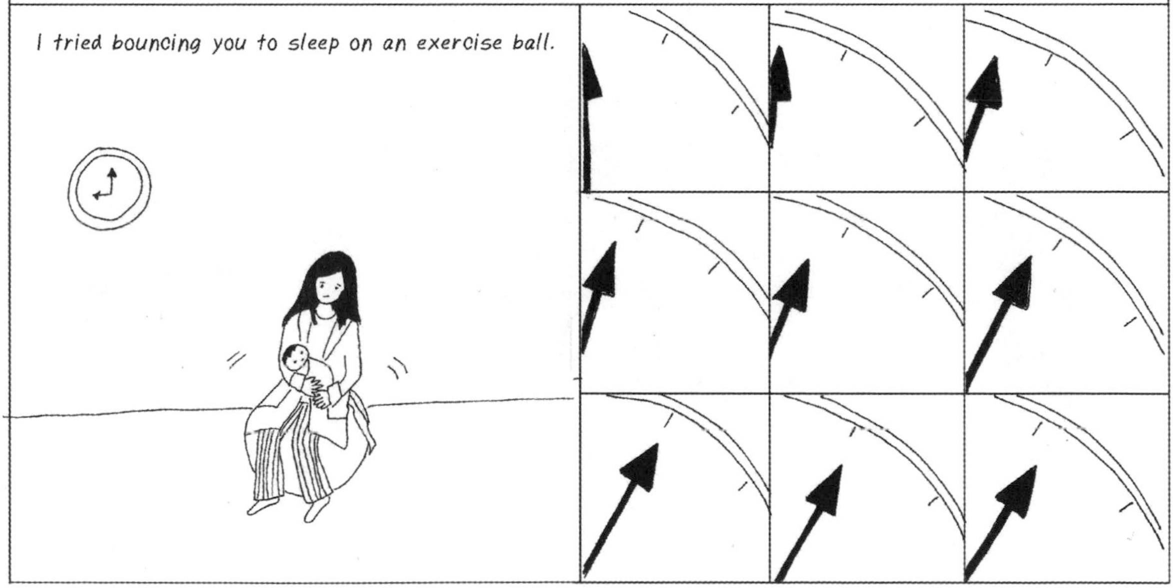
I tried bouncing you to sleep on an exercise ball.

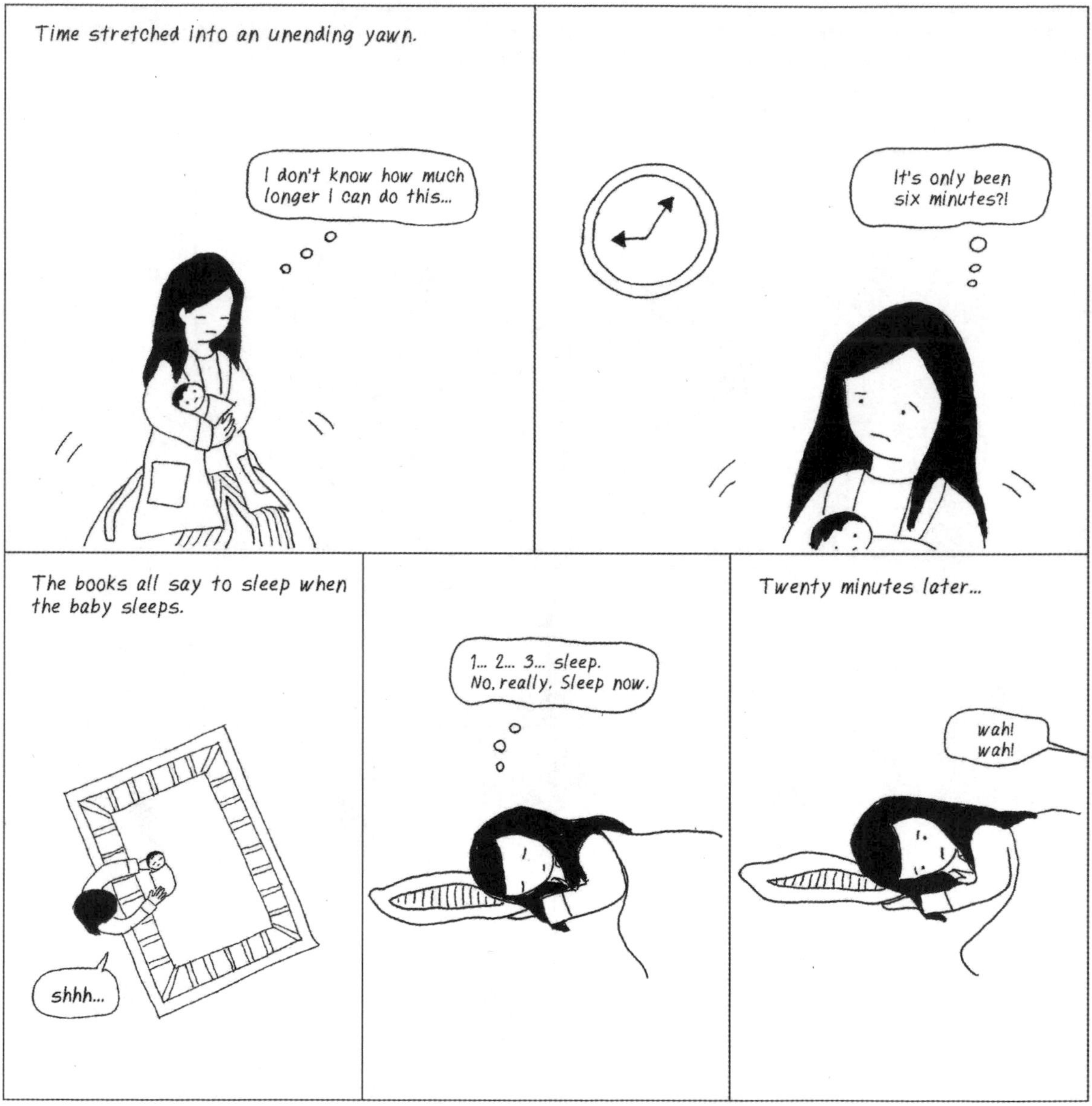
Time stretched into an unending yawn.
I don't know how much longer I can do this...
It's only been six minutes?!
The books all say to sleep when the baby sleeps.
shhh...
1... 2... 3... sleep. No, really. Sleep now.
Twenty minutes later...
wah! wah!

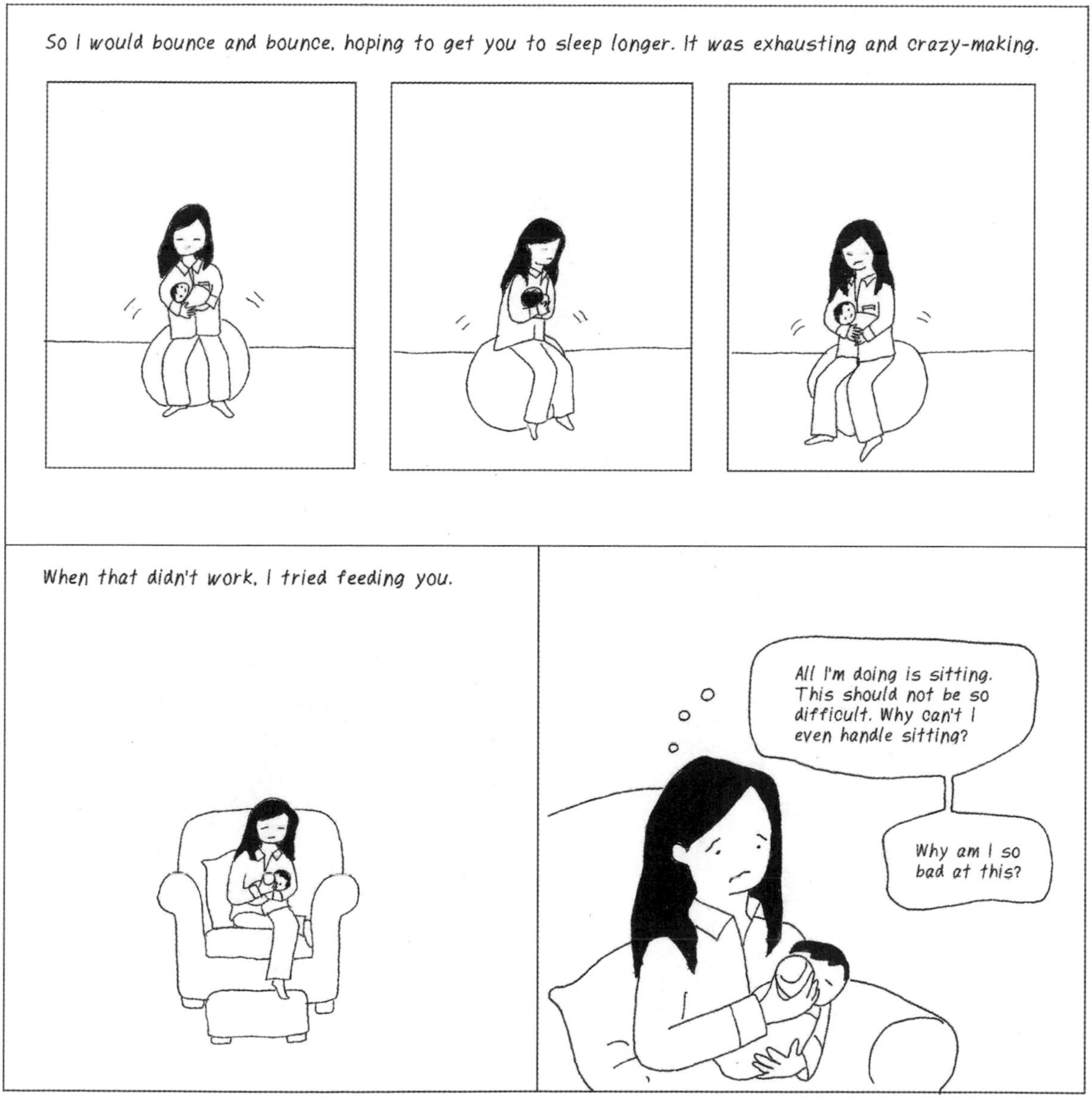
So I would bounce and bounce, hoping to get you to sleep longer. It was exhausting and crazy-making.
When that didn't work, I tried feeding you.
All I'm doing is sitting. This should not be so difficult. Why can't I even handle sitting?
Why am I so bad at this?

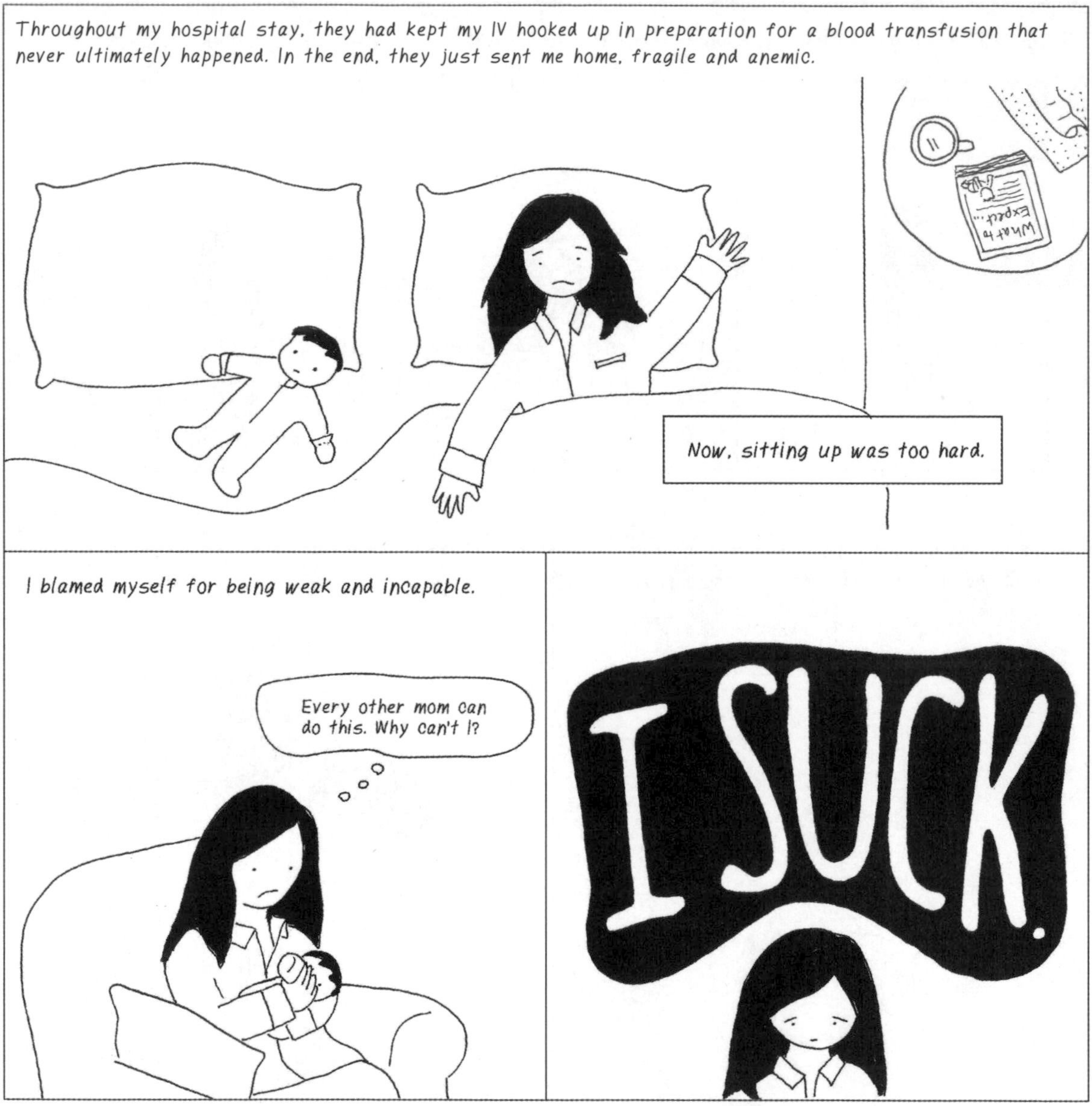
Throughout my hospital stay, they had kept my IV hooked up in preparation for a blood transfusion that never ultimately happened. In the end, they just sent me home, fragile and anemic.
What to Expect...
Now, sitting up was too hard.
I blamed myself for being weak and incapable.
Every other mom can do this. Why can't I?
I SUCK.

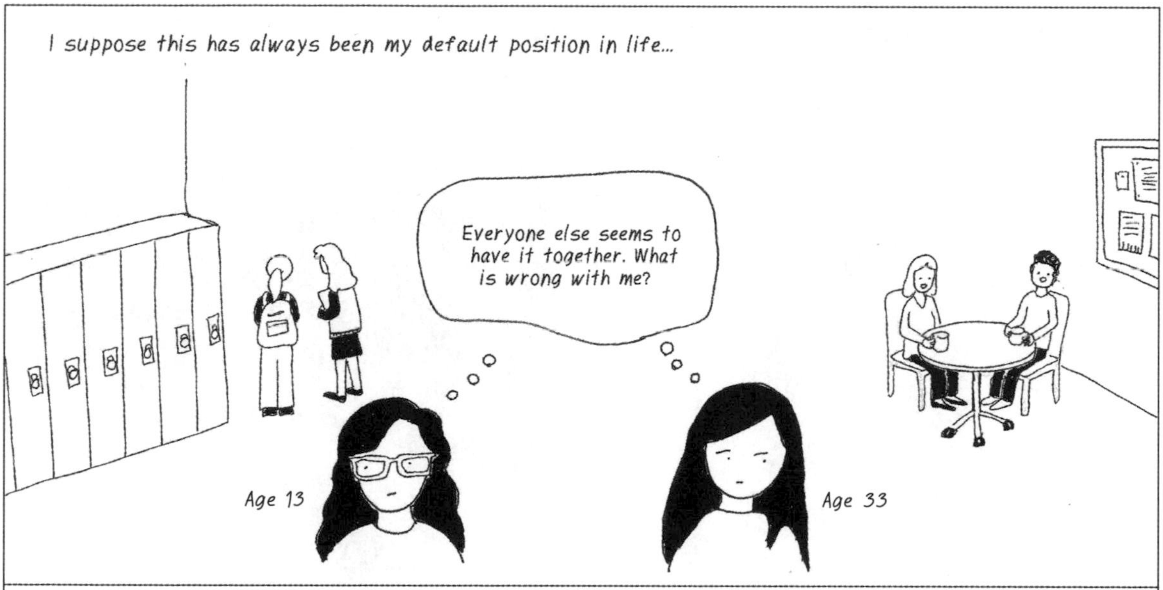
I suppose this has always been my default position in life...
Everyone else seems to have it together. What is wrong with me?
Age 13
Age 33

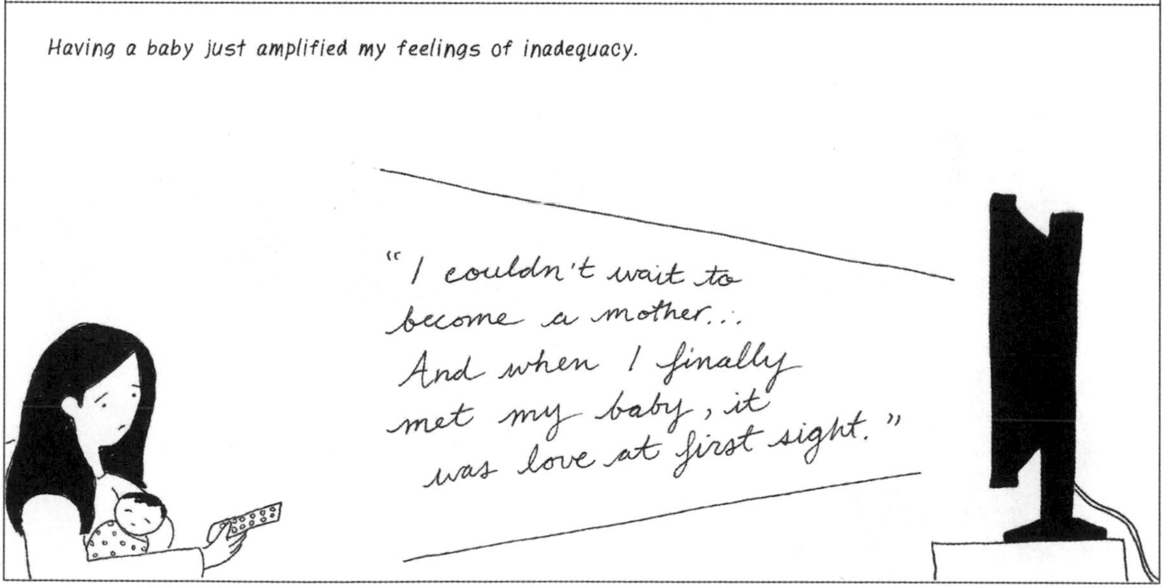
Having a baby just amplified my feelings of inadequacy.
"I couldn't wait to become a mother... And when I finally met my baby, it was love at first sight."

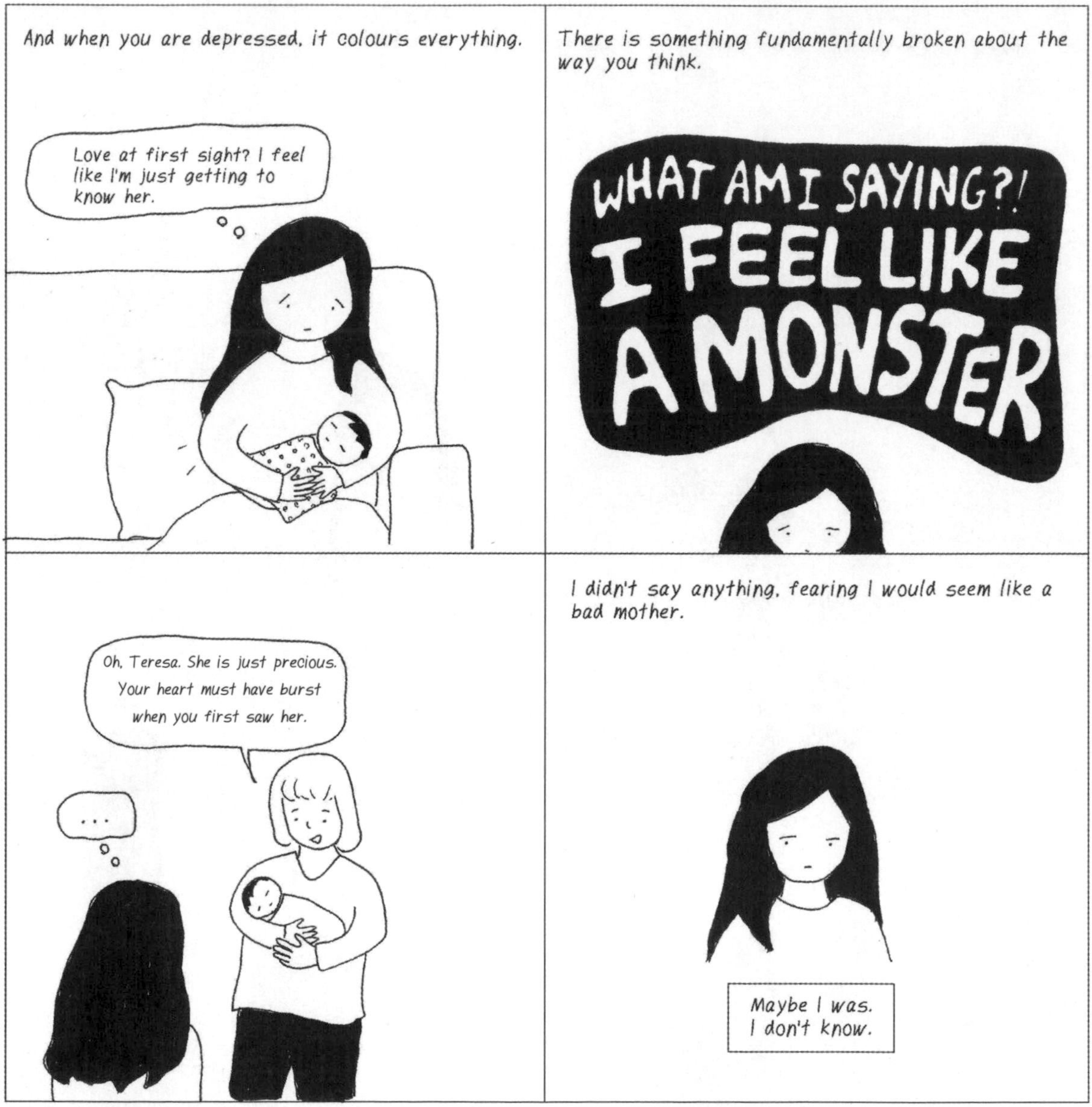
And when you are depressed, it colours everything.
Love at first sight? I feel like I'm just getting to know her.
There is something fundamentally broken about the way you think.
WHAT AM I SAYING?! I FEEL LIKE A MONSTER
Oh, Teresa. She is just precious. Your heart must have burst when you first saw her.
...
I didn't say anything, fearing I would seem like a bad mother.
Maybe I was. I don't know.

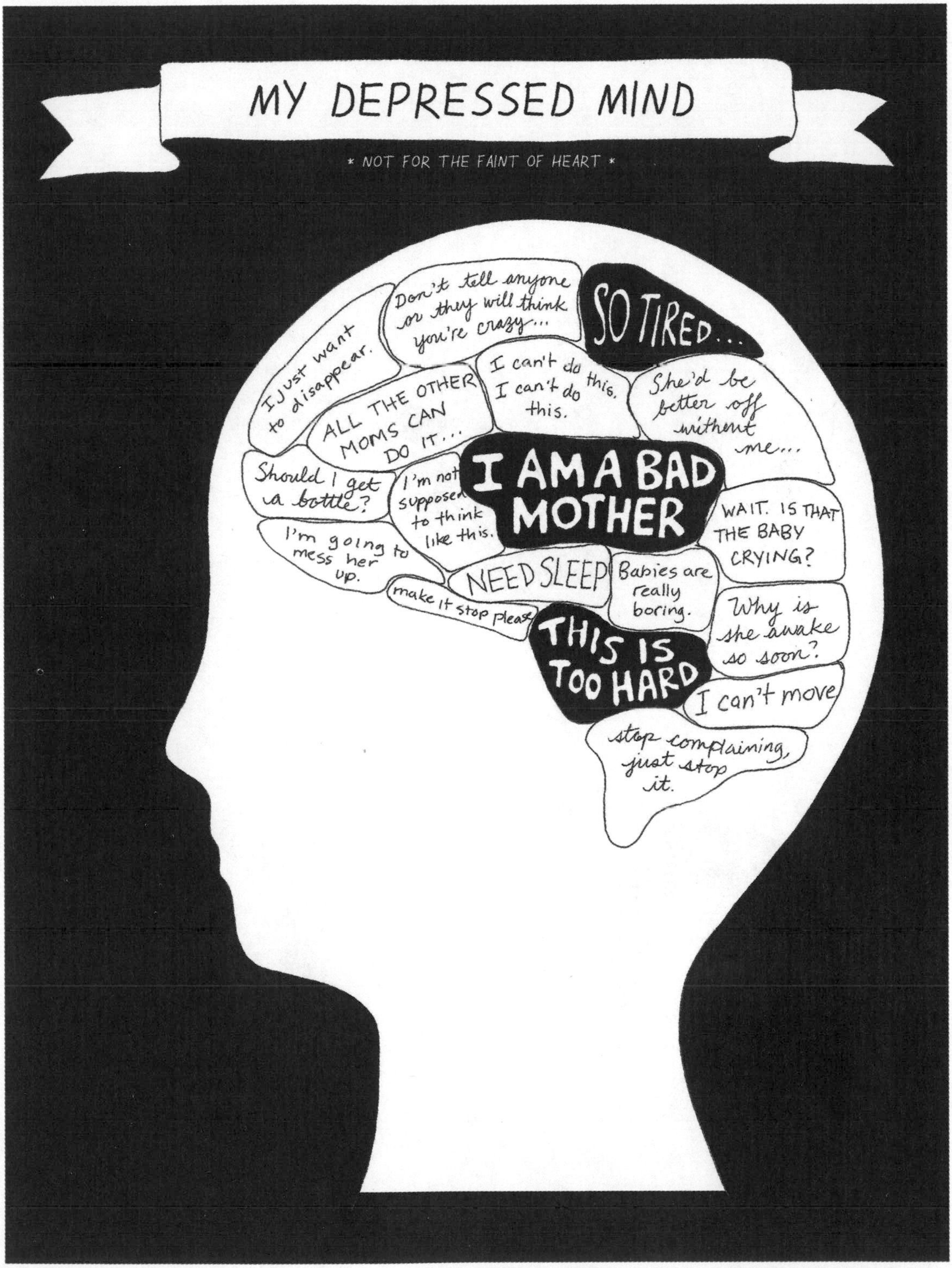
MY DEPRESSED MIND
* NOT FOR THE FAINT OF HEART *
I just want to disappear.
Don't tell anyone or they will think you're crazy...
SO TIRED...
ALL THE OTHER MOMS CAN DO IT...
I can't do this. I can't do this.
She'd be better off without me...
Should I get a bottle?
I'm not supposed to think like this.
I AM A BAD MOTHER
WAIT. IS THAT THE BABY CRYING?
I'm going to mess her up.
NEED SLEEP
Babies are really boring.
make it stop please
THIS IS TOO HARD
Why is she awake so soon?
I can't move
stop complaining, just stop it.

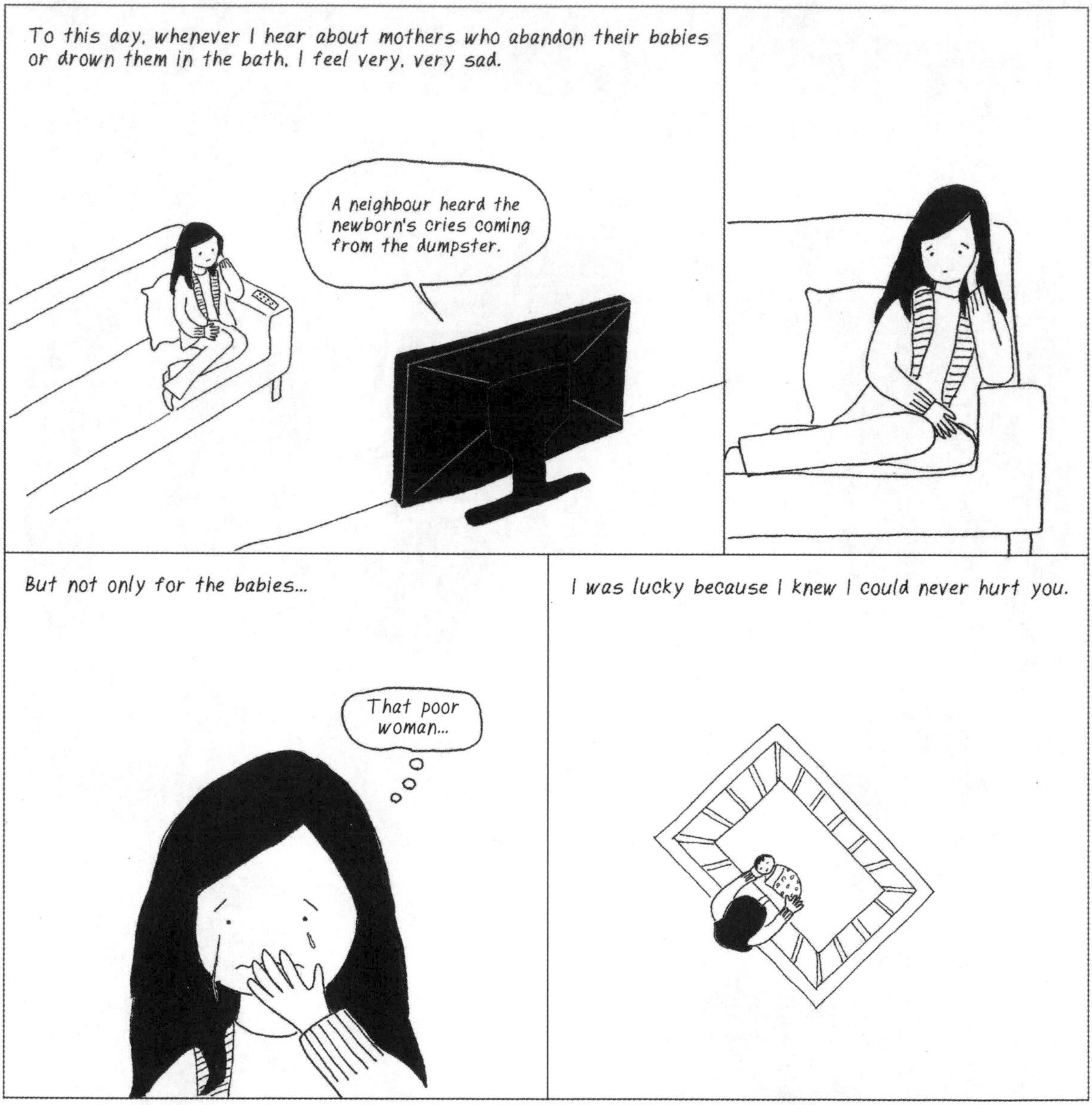
To this day, whenever I hear about mothers who abandon their babies or drown them in the bath, I feel very, very sad.
A neighbour heard the newborn's cries coming from the dumpster.
But not only for the babies...
That poor woman...
I was lucky because I knew I could never hurt you.

But I understood what it was like to feel trapped. I could never go back to the life I'd had.
And my new life was full of worry, fatigue and disconnectedness.
I fantasized about leaving, just getting in the car and driving away.
She'd be better off without me.
Or simply going to sleep forever.

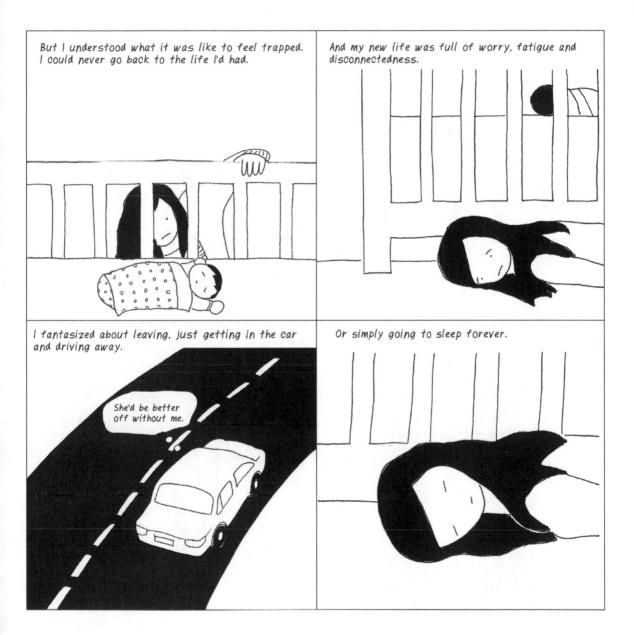

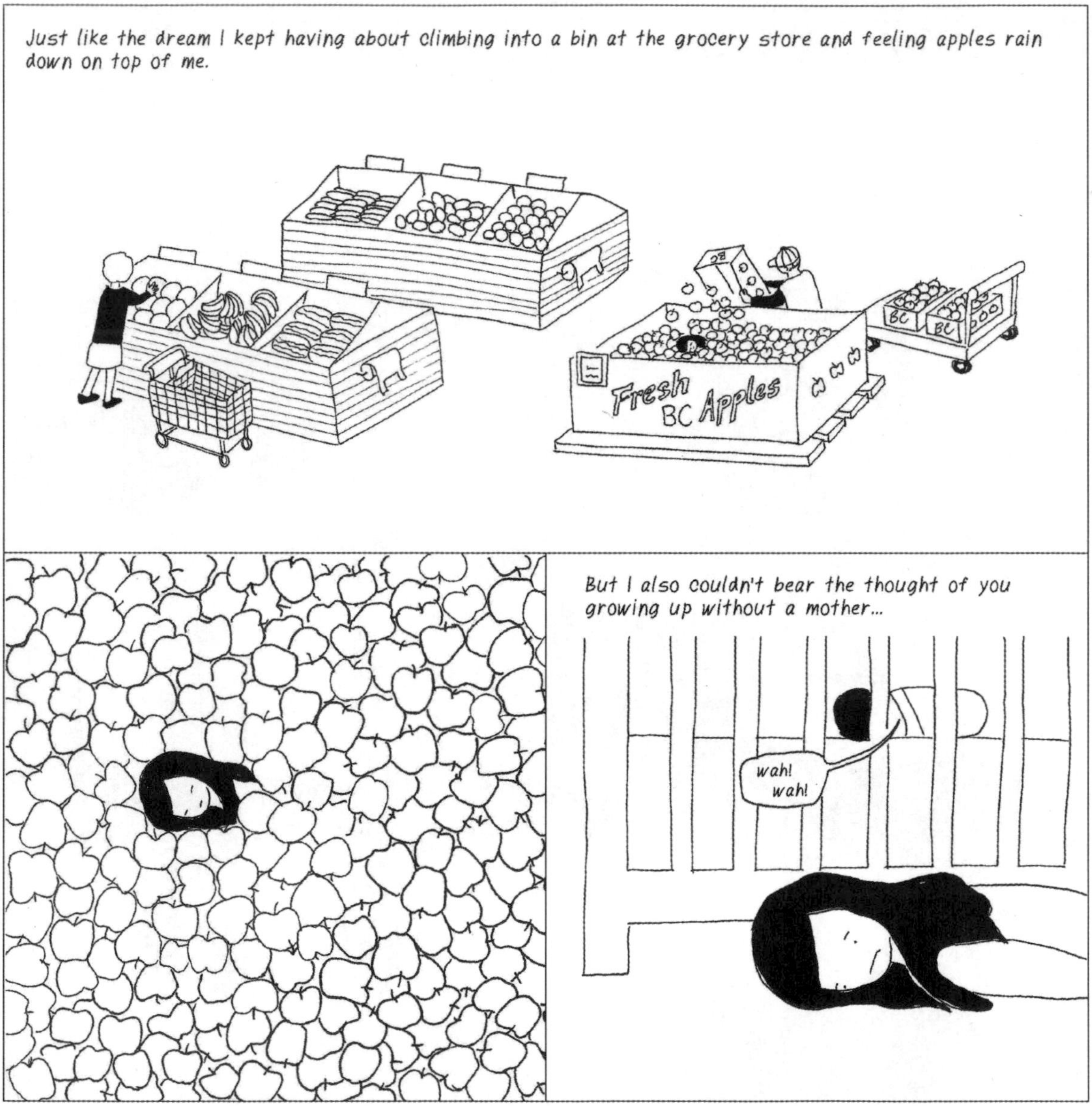
Just like the dream I kept having about climbing into a bin at the grocery store and feeling apples rain down on top of me.
Fresh BC Apples
But I also couldn't bear the thought of you growing up without a mother...
wah! wah!

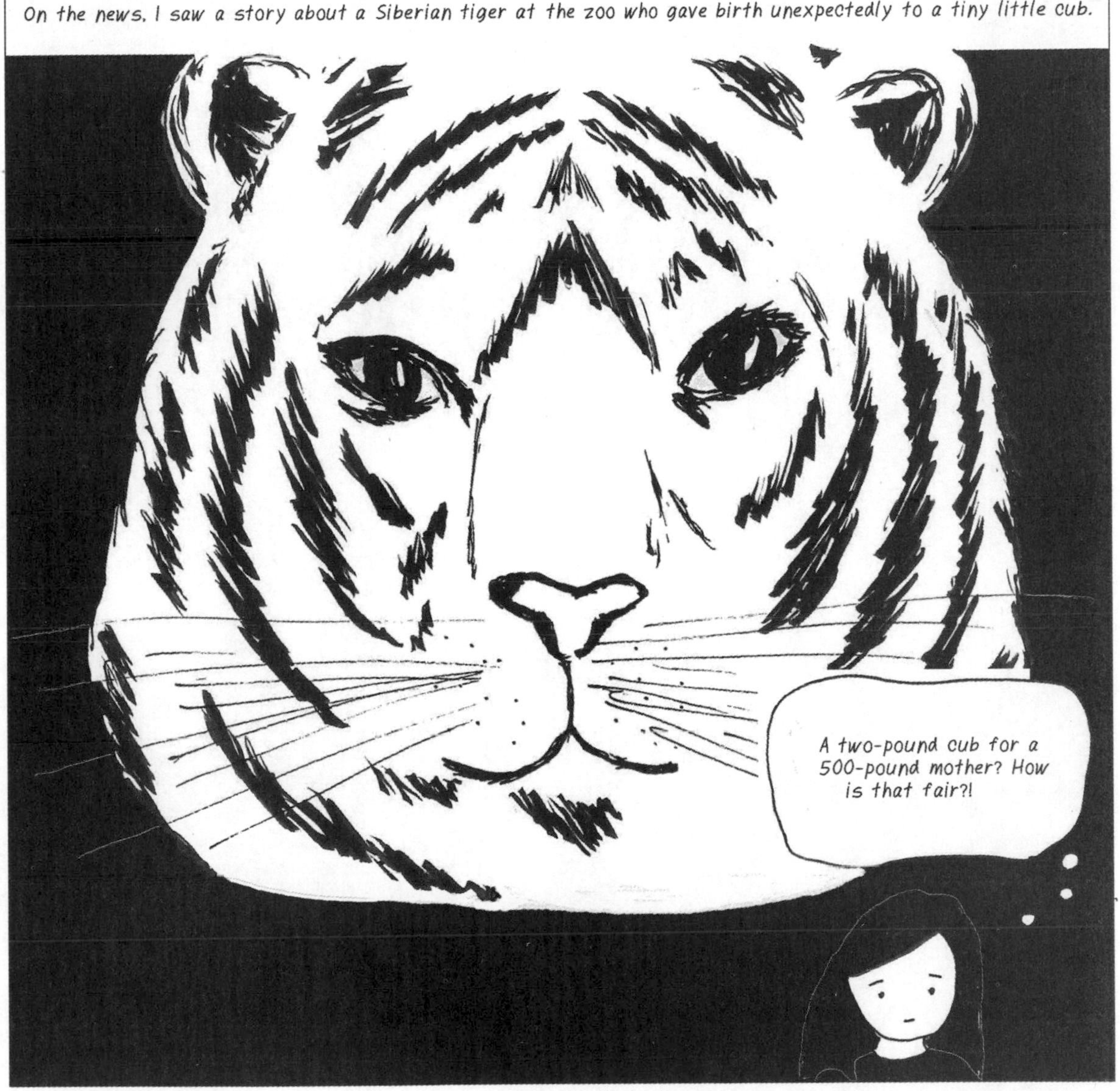
On the news, I saw a story about a Siberian tiger at the zoo who gave birth unexpectedly to a tiny little cub.
A two-pound cub for a 500-pound mother? How is that fair?!

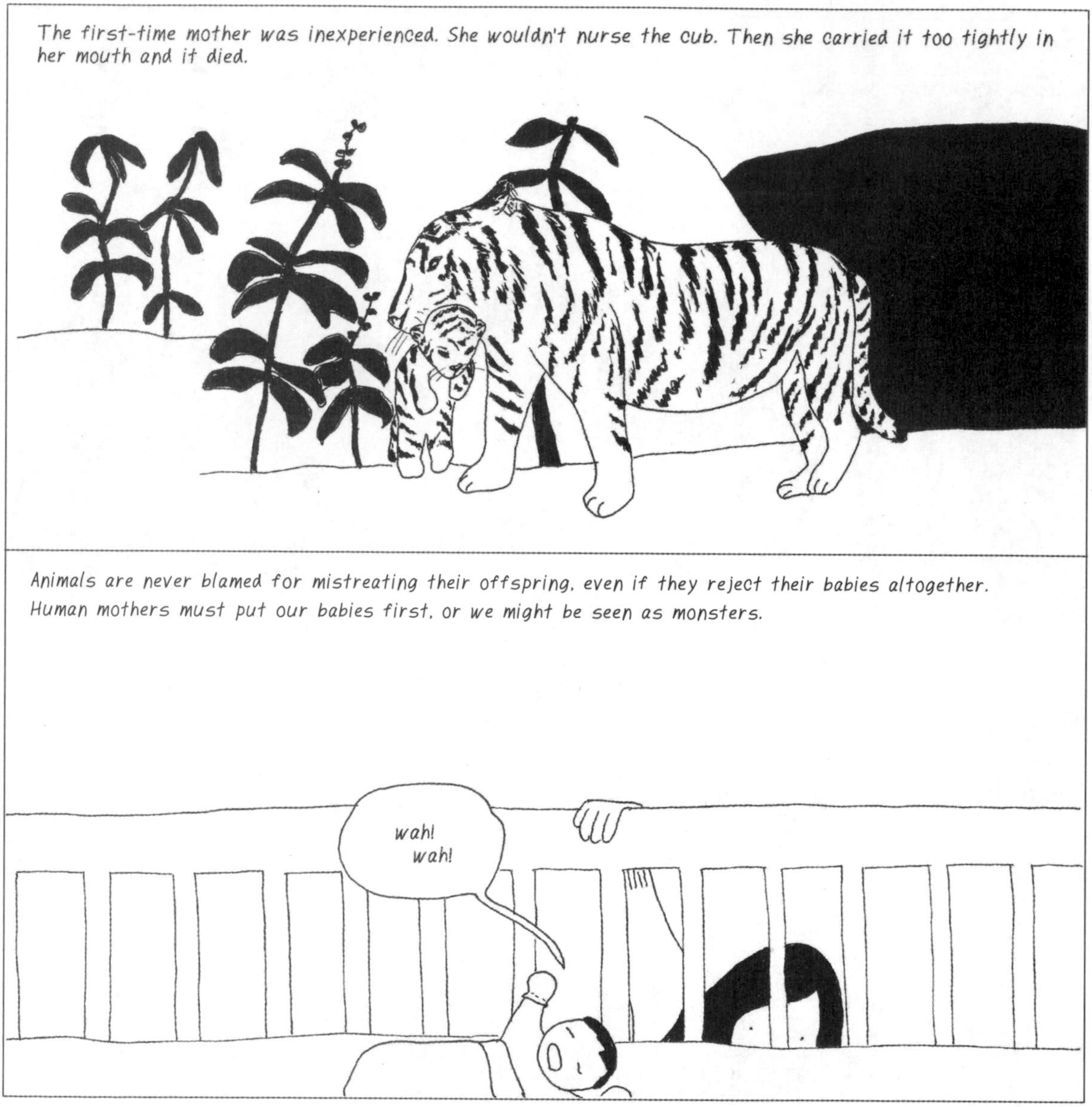
The first-time mother was inexperienced. She wouldn't nurse the cub. Then she carried it too tightly in her mouth and it died.
Animals are never blamed for mistreating their offspring, even if they reject their babies altogether. Human mothers must put our babies first, or we might be seen as monsters.
wah! wah!

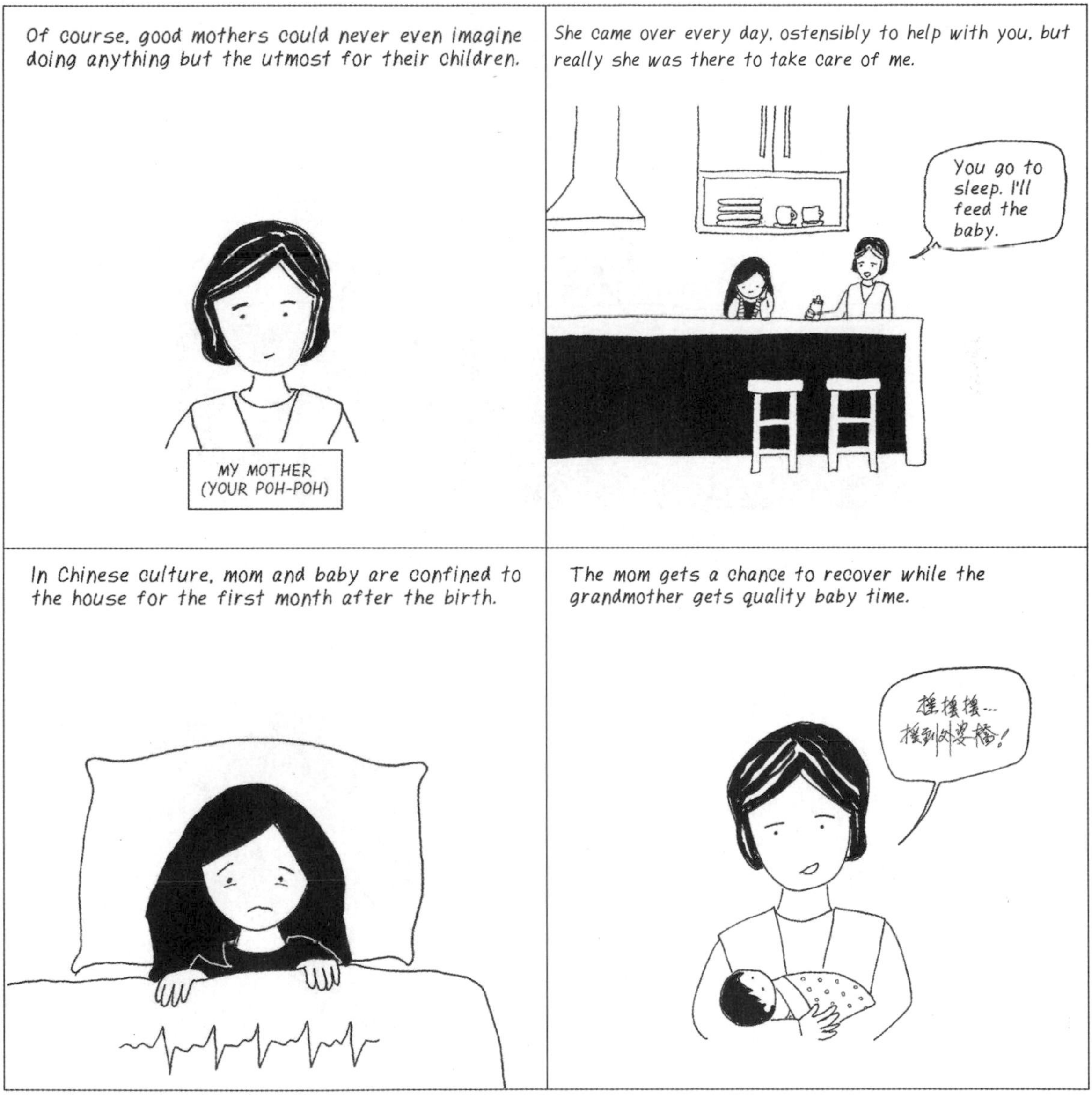
Of course, good mothers could never even imagine doing anything but the utmost for their children.
MY MOTHER (YOUR POH-POH)
She came over every day, ostensibly to help with you, but really she was there to take care of me.
You go to sleep. I'll feed the baby.
In Chinese culture, mom and baby are confined to the house for the first month after the birth.
The mom gets a chance to recover while the grandmother gets quality baby time.
搖搖搖...
搖到外婆橋!

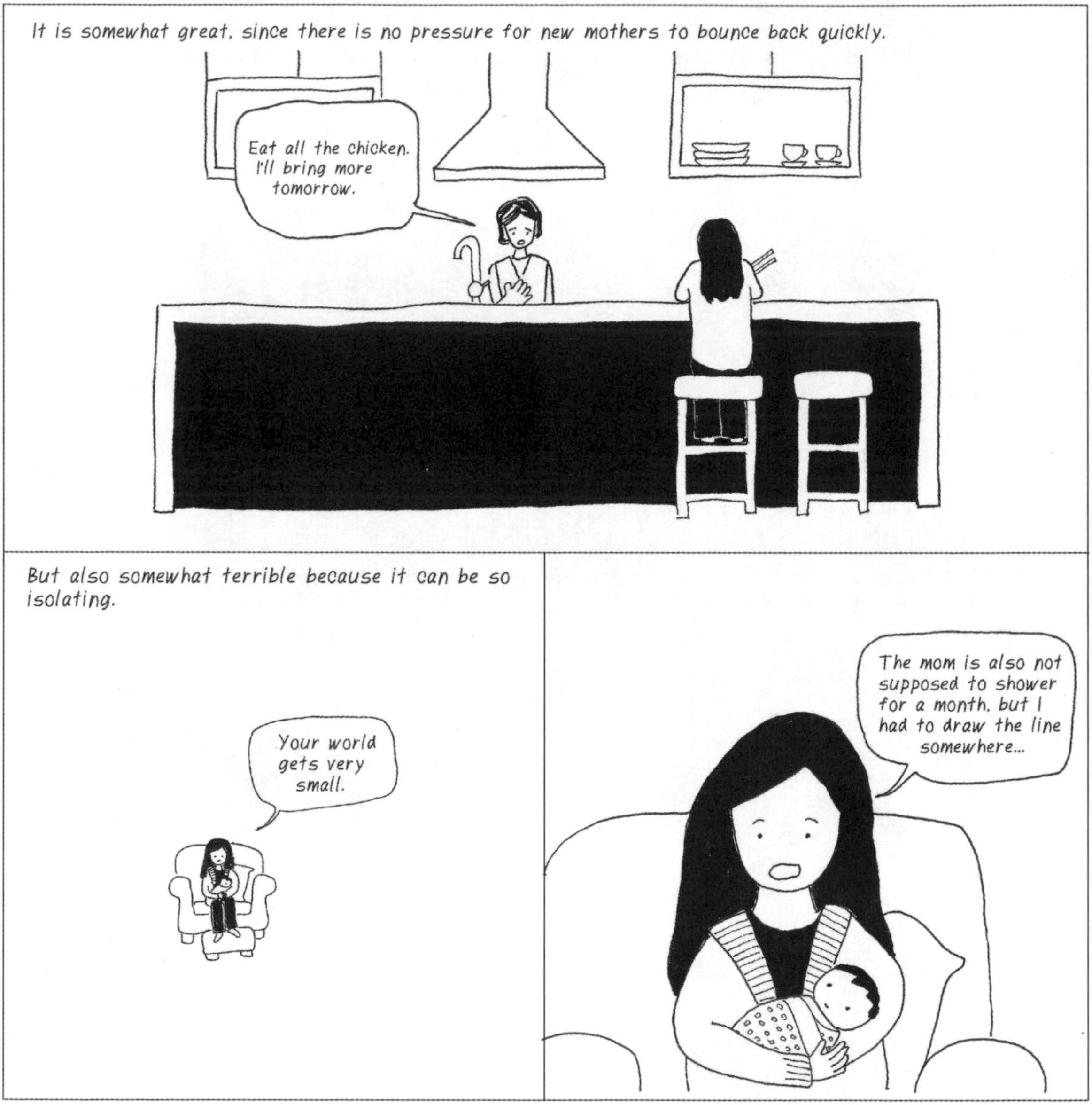
It is somewhat great, since there is no pressure for new mothers to bounce back quickly.
Eat all the chicken. I'll bring more tomorrow.
But also somewhat terrible because it can be so isolating.
Your world gets very small.
The mom is also not supposed to shower for a month, but I had to draw the line somewhere...

CHINESE POSTPARTUM FOOD

* NOT FOR THE FAINT OF HEART *

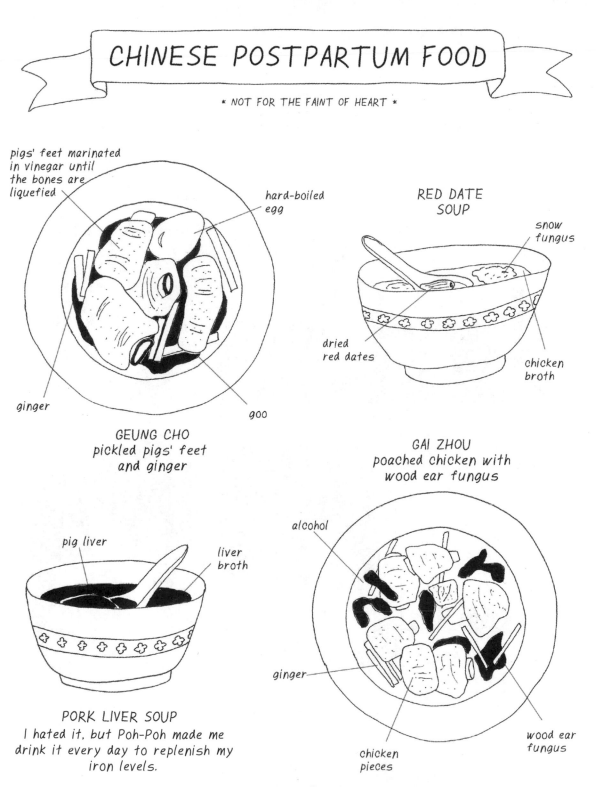

pigs' feet marinated in vinegar until the bones are liquefied

hard-boiled egg

RED DATE SOUP

snow fungus

dried red dates

chicken broth

ginger

goo

GEUNG CHO
pickled pigs' feet and ginger

GAI ZHOU
poached chicken with wood ear fungus

pig liver

liver broth

alcohol

ginger

chicken pieces

wood ear fungus

PORK LIVER SOUP
I hated it, but Poh-Poh made me drink it every day to replenish my iron levels.

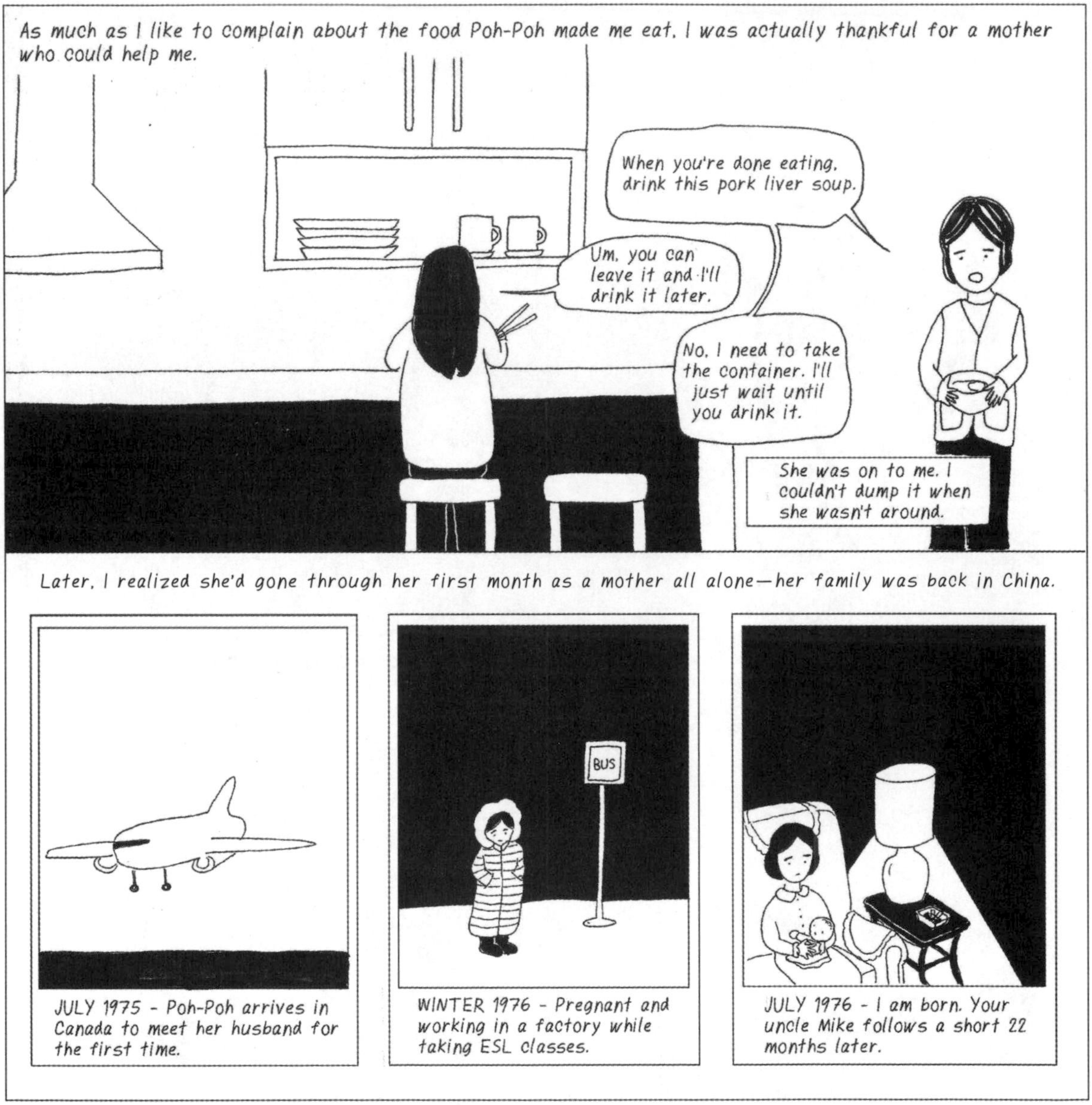
As much as I like to complain about the food Poh-Poh made me eat, I was actually thankful for a mother who could help me.
When you're done eating, drink this pork liver soup.
Um, you can leave it and I'll drink it later.
No, I need to take the container. I'll just wait until you drink it.
She was on to me. I couldn't dump it when she wasn't around.
Later, I realized she'd gone through her first month as a mother all alone—her family was back in China.
JULY 1975 - Poh-Poh arrives in Canada to meet her husband for the first time.
BUS
WINTER 1976 - Pregnant and working in a factory while taking ESL classes.
JULY 1976 - I am born. Your uncle Mike follows a short 22 months later.

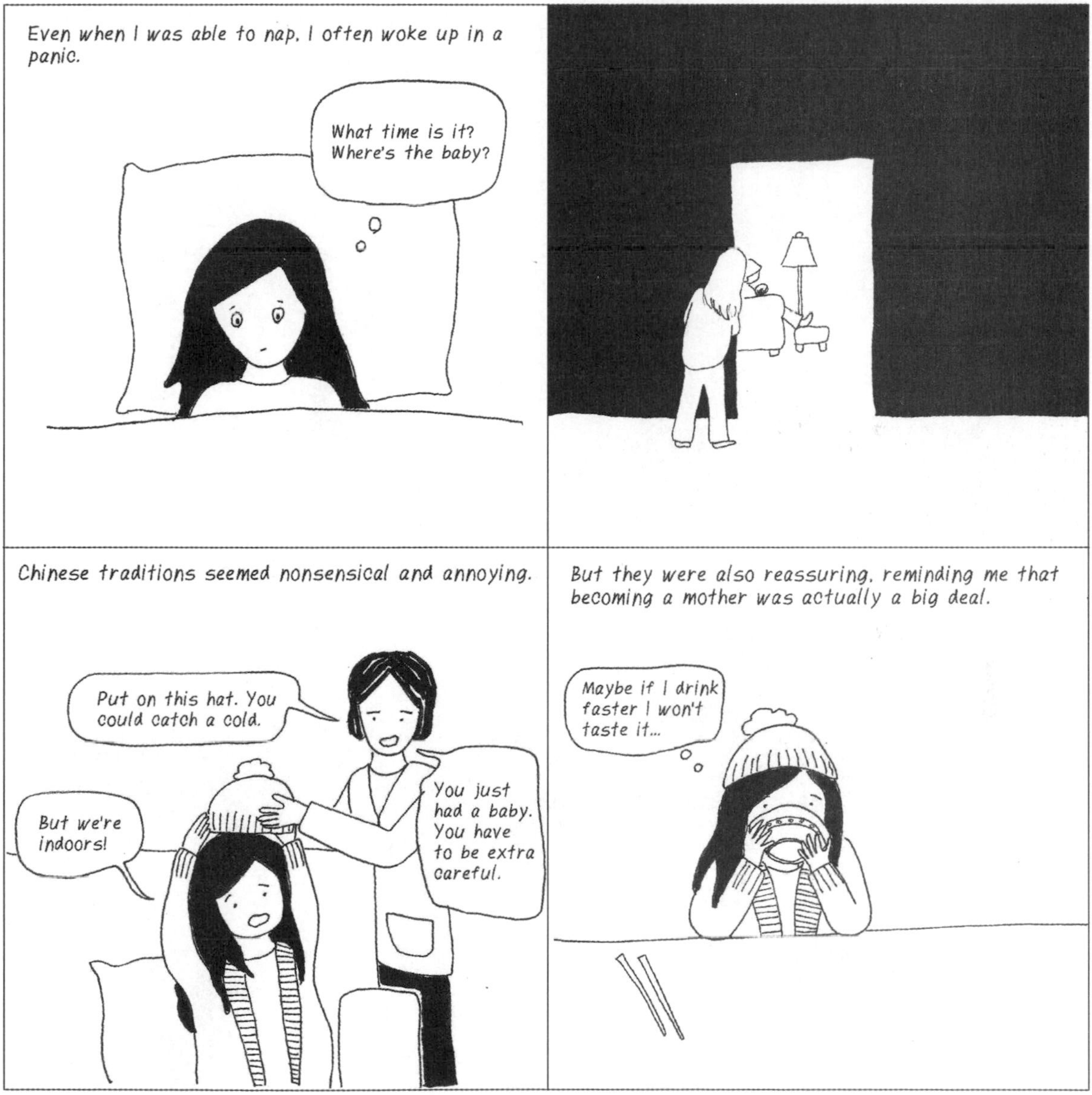
Even when I was able to nap, I often woke up in a panic.
What time is it? Where's the baby?
Chinese traditions seemed nonsensical and annoying.
Put on this hat. You could catch a cold.
But we're indoors!
You just had a baby. You have to be extra careful.
But they were also reassuring, reminding me that becoming a mother was actually a big deal.
Maybe if I drink faster I won't taste it...

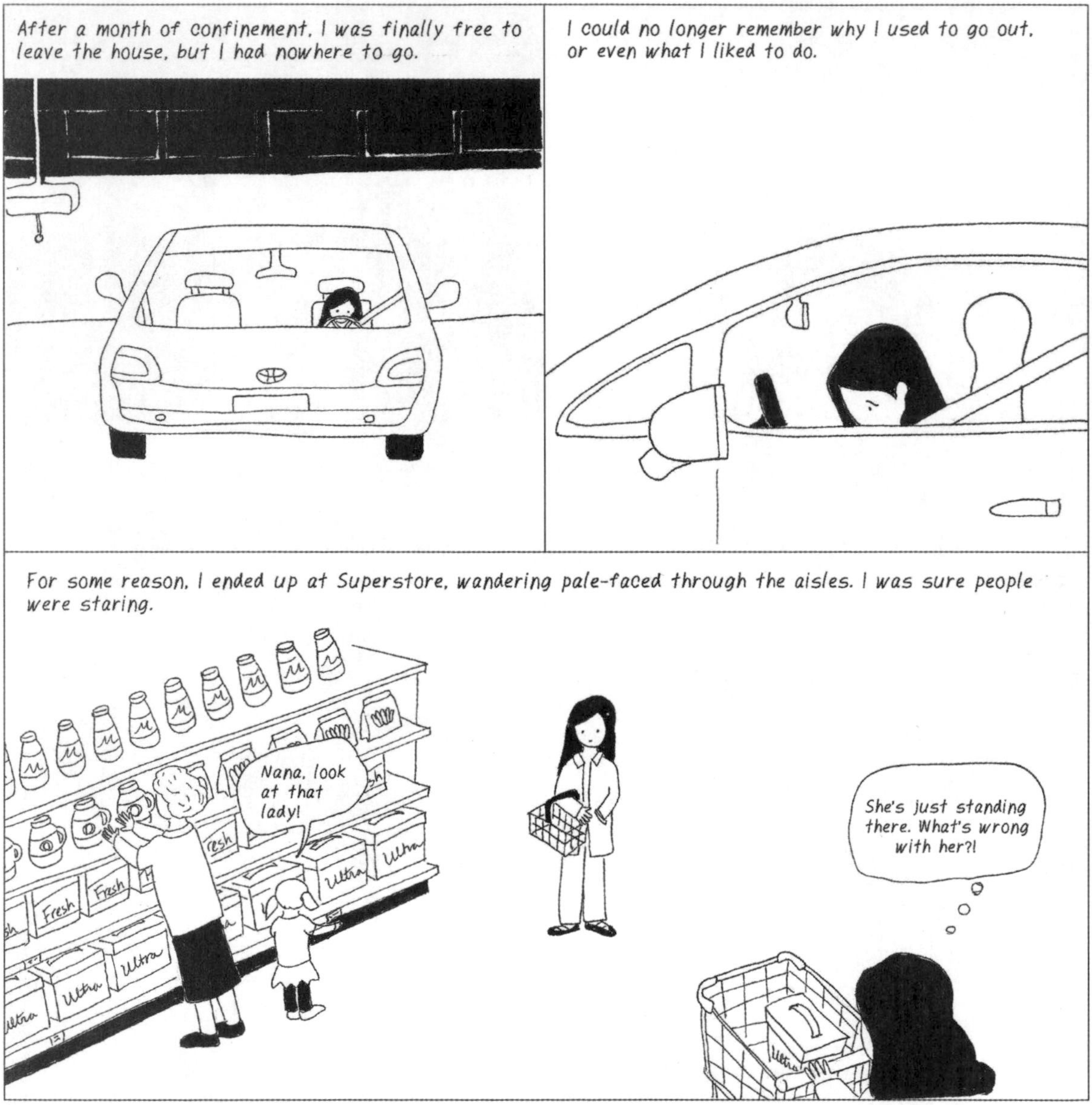
After a month of confinement, I was finally free to leave the house, but I had nowhere to go.
I could no longer remember why I used to go out, or even what I liked to do.
For some reason, I ended up at Superstore, wandering pale-faced through the aisles. I was sure people were staring.
Nana, look at that lady!
She's just standing there. What's wrong with her?!
Fresh
Ultra

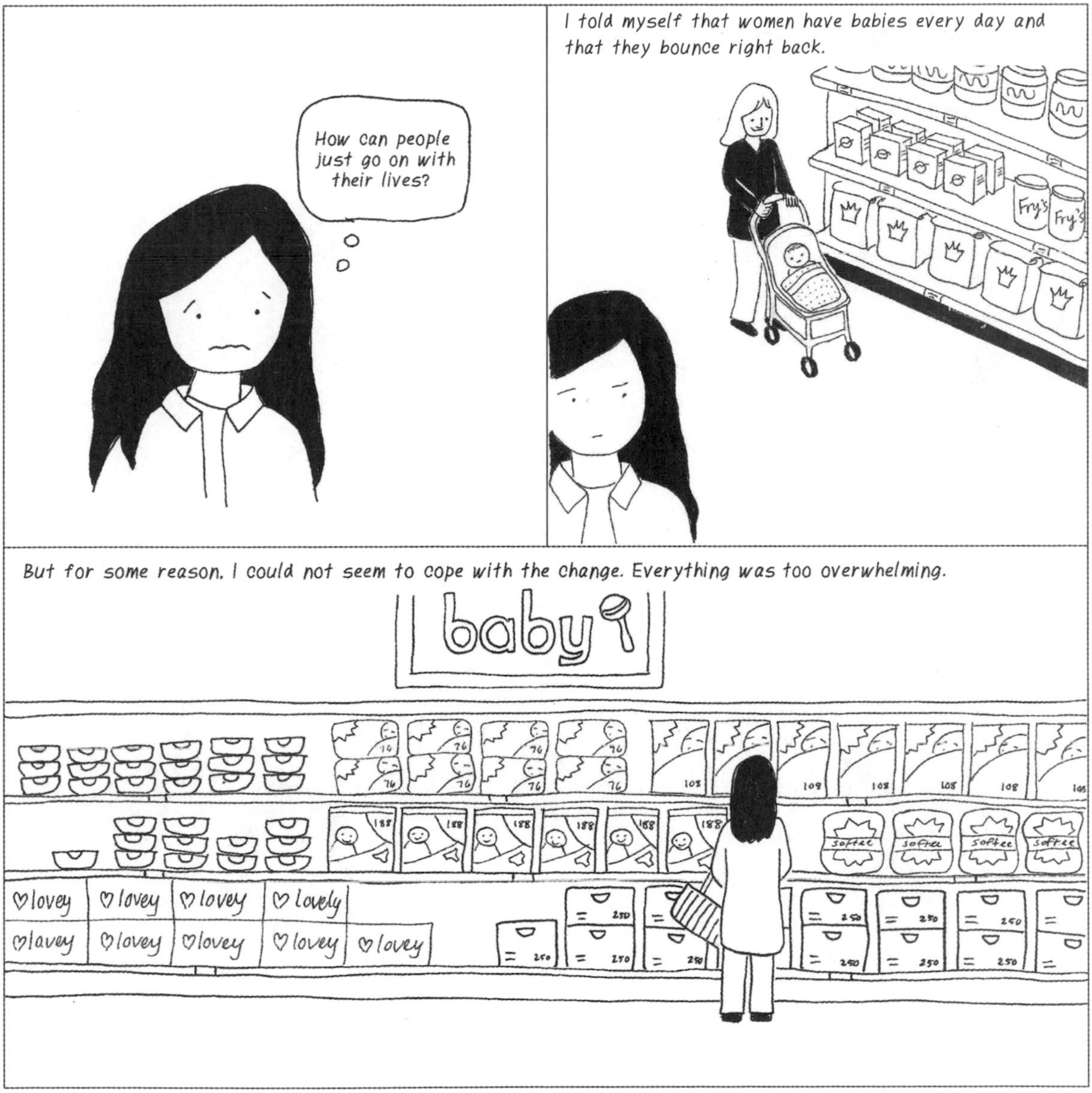
How can people just go on with their lives?
I told myself that women have babies every day and that they bounce right back.
Fry's
Fry's
But for some reason, I could not seem to cope with the change. Everything was too overwhelming.
baby
softee
softee
softee
softee
lovey
lovey
lovey
lovely
lavey
lovey
lovey
lovey
lovey

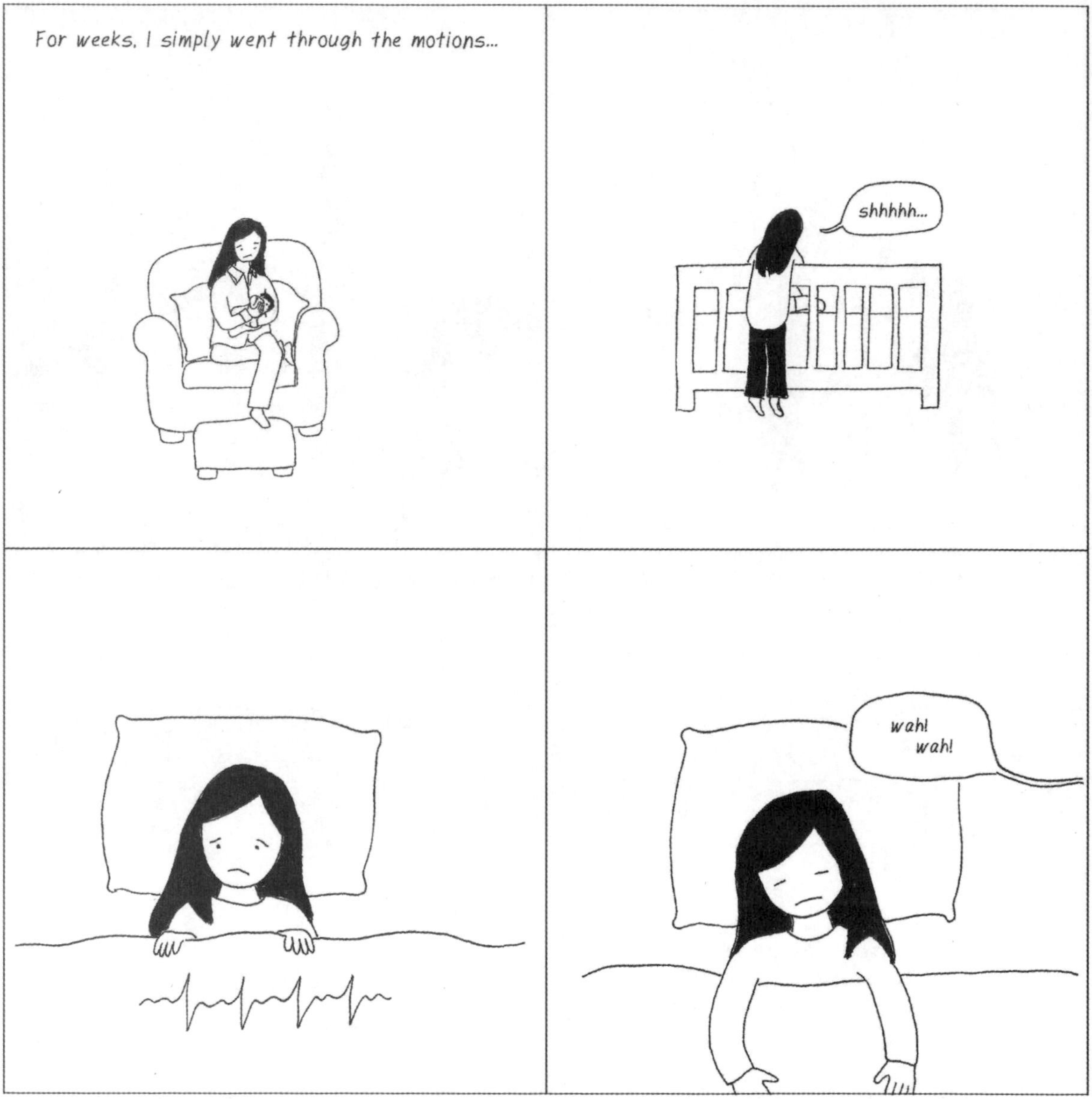
For weeks, I simply went through the motions...
shhhhh...
wah!
wah!

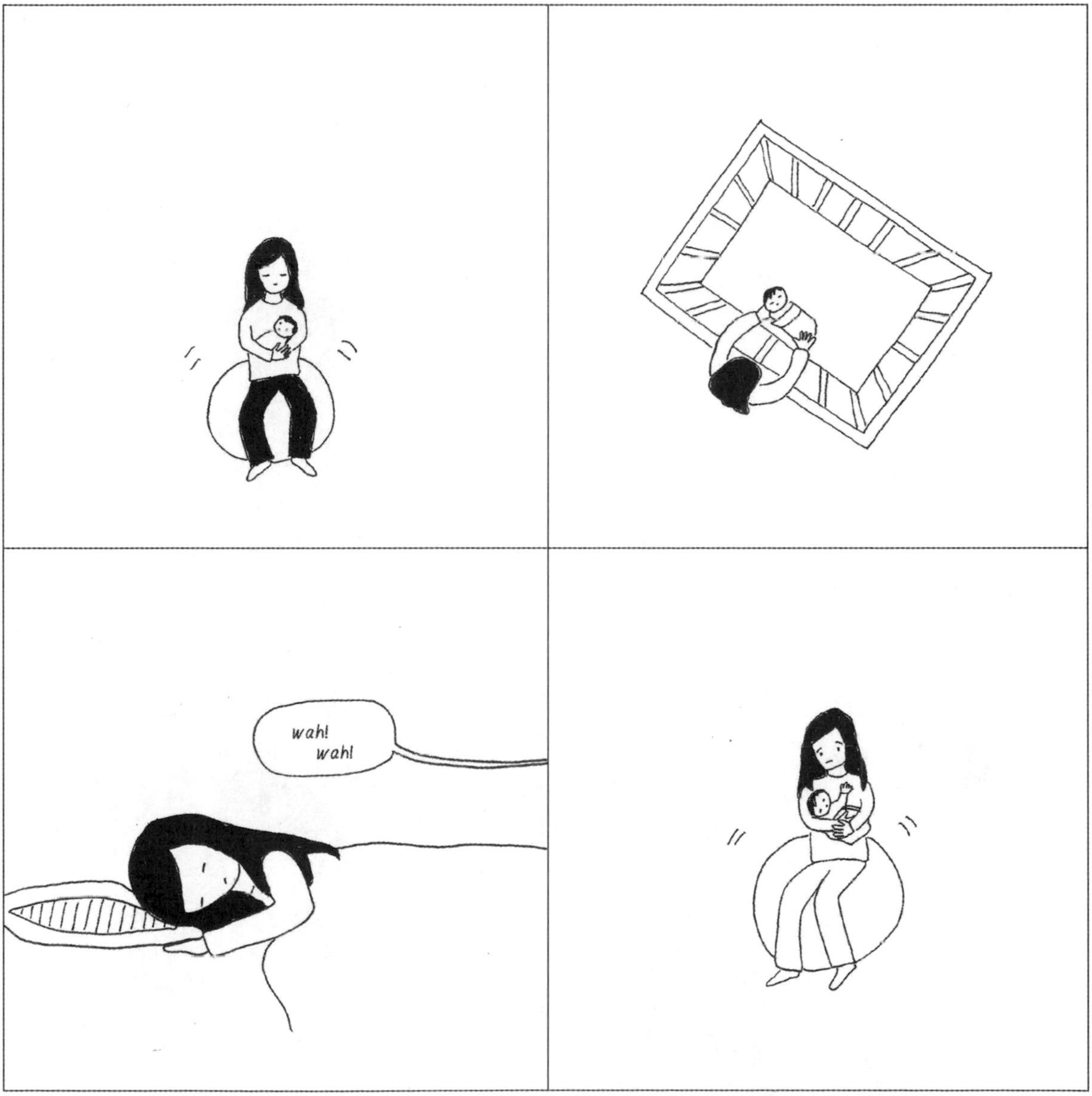
wah! wah!

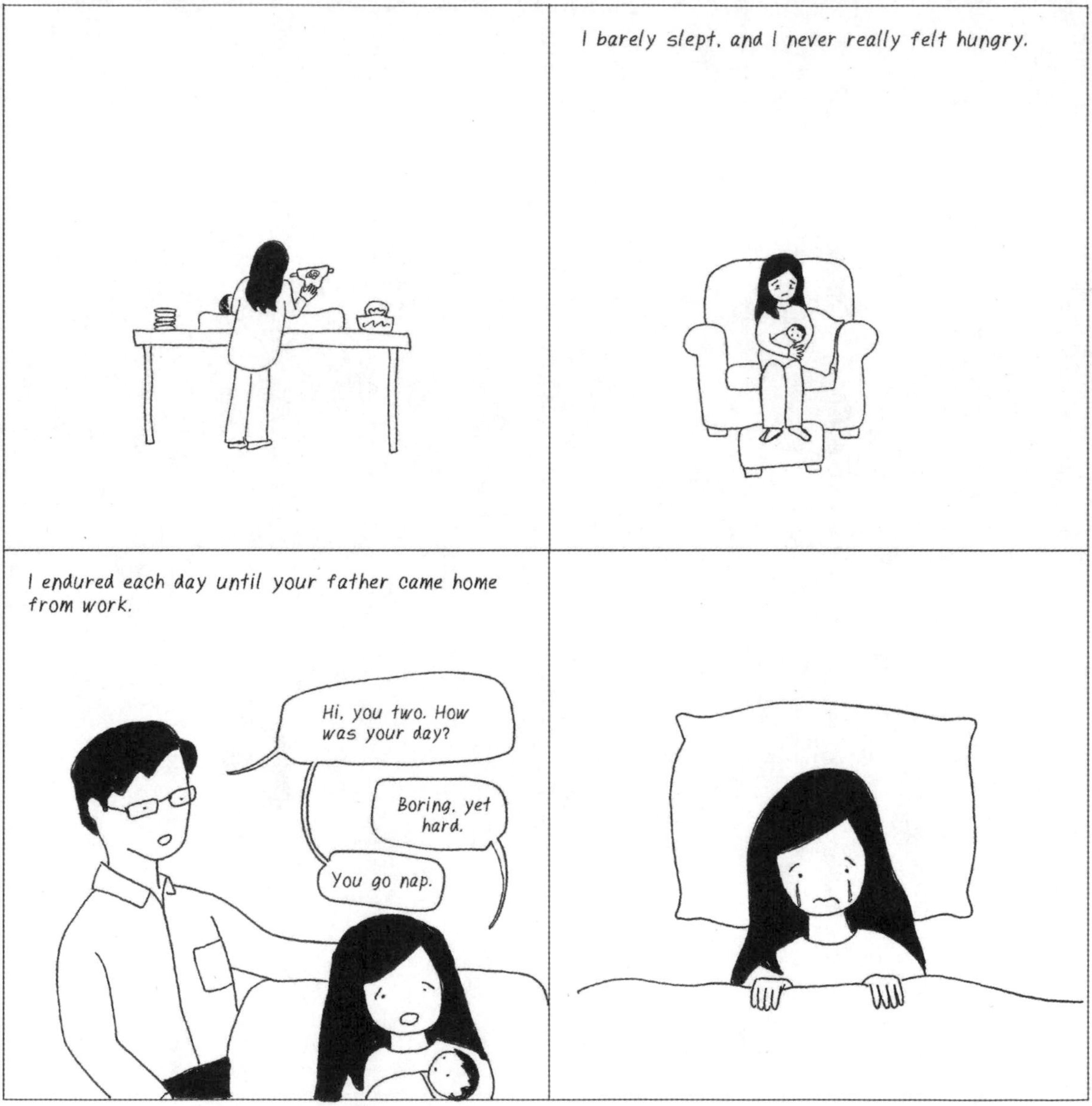
I barely slept, and I never really felt hungry.
I endured each day until your father came home from work.
Hi, you two. How was your day?
Boring, yet hard.
You go nap.

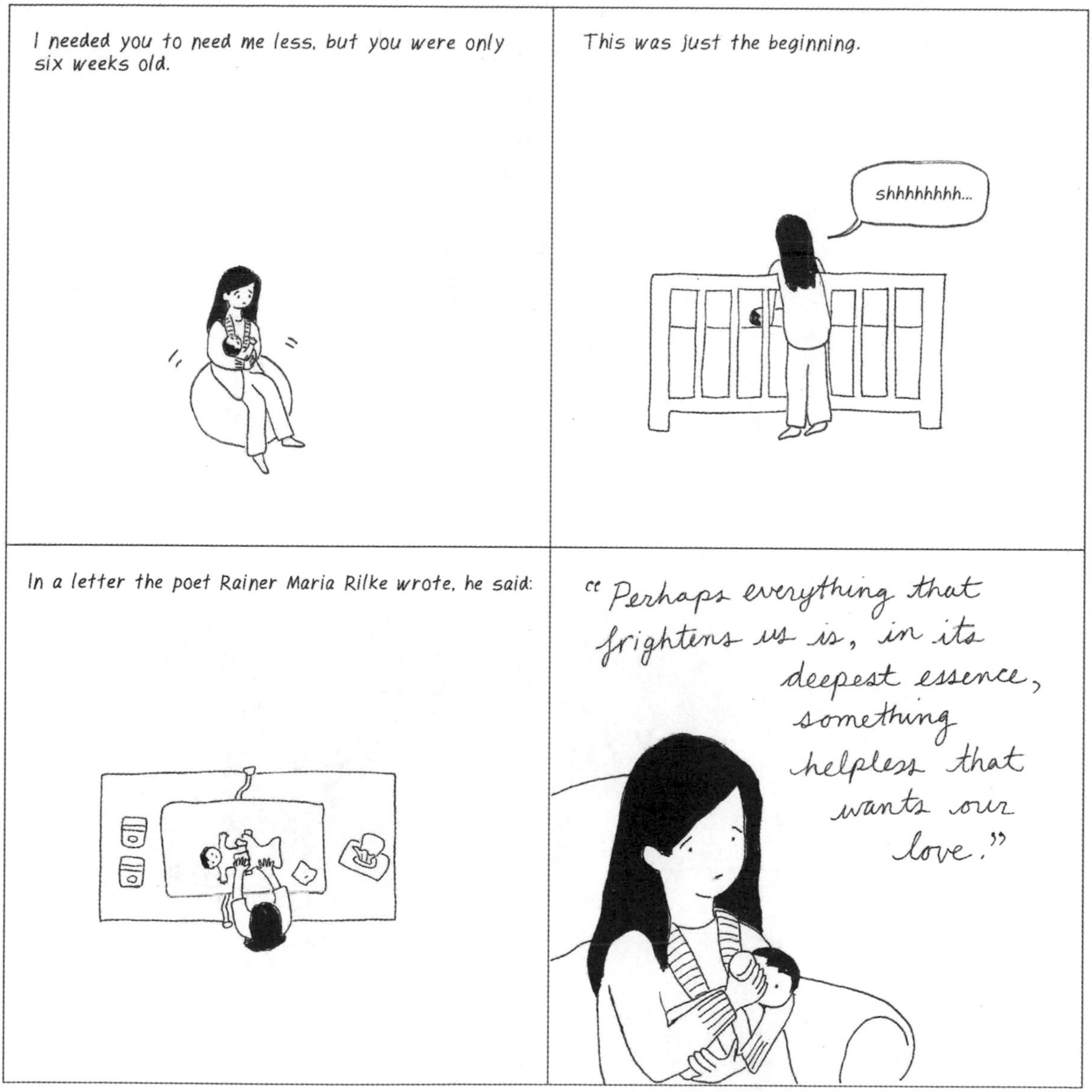
I needed you to need me less, but you were only six weeks old.
This was just the beginning.
shhhhhhhh...
In a letter the poet Rainer Maria Rilke wrote, he said:
"Perhaps everything that frightens us is, in its deepest essence, something helpless that wants our love."

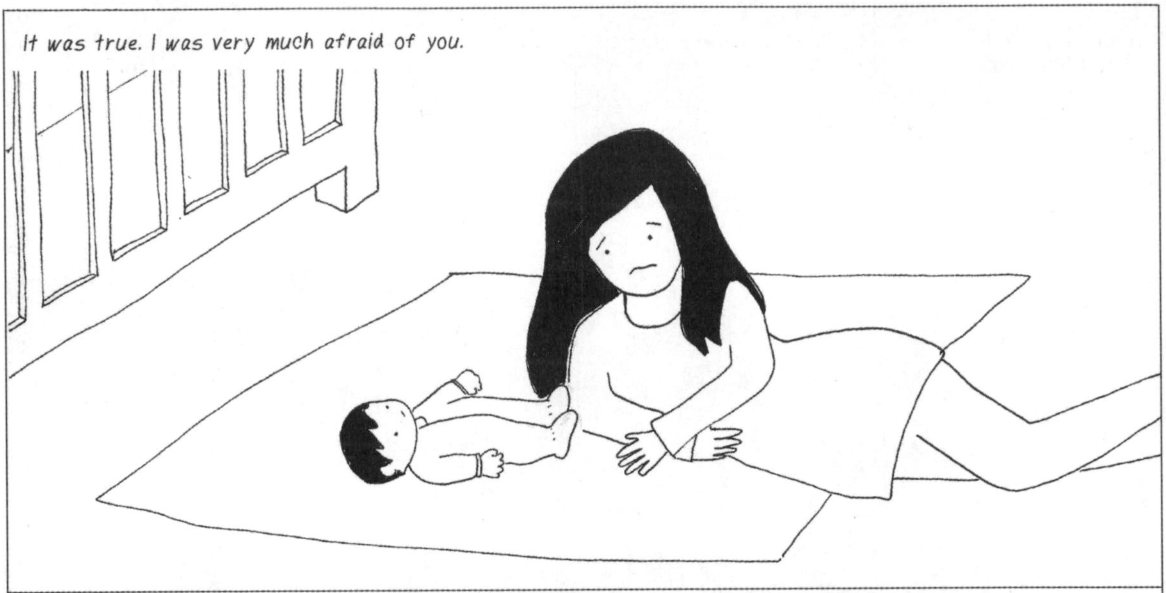
It was true. I was very much afraid of you.

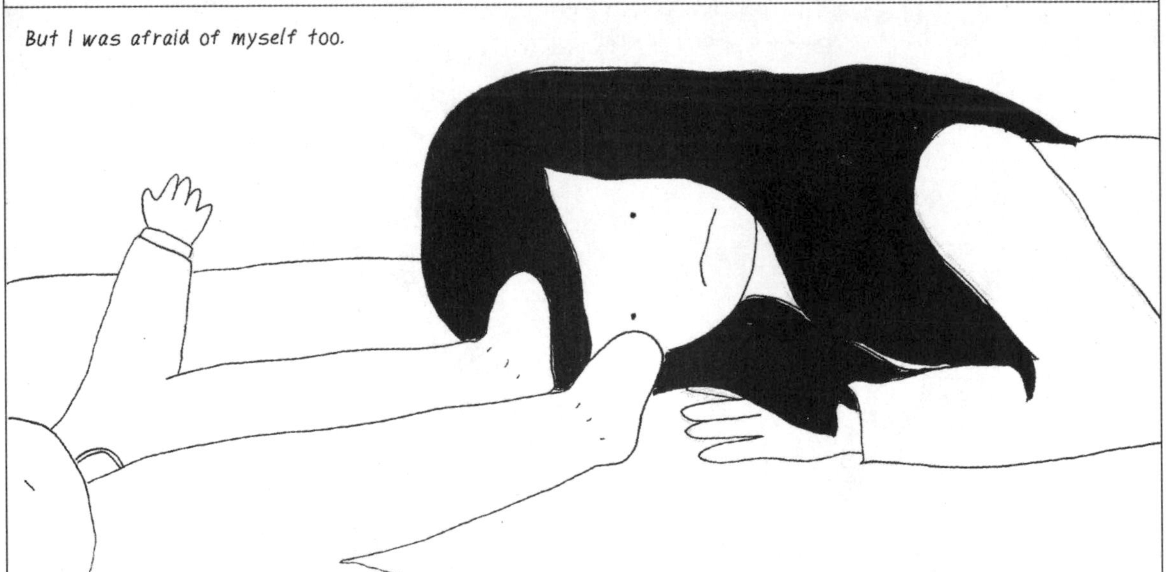
But I was afraid of myself too.

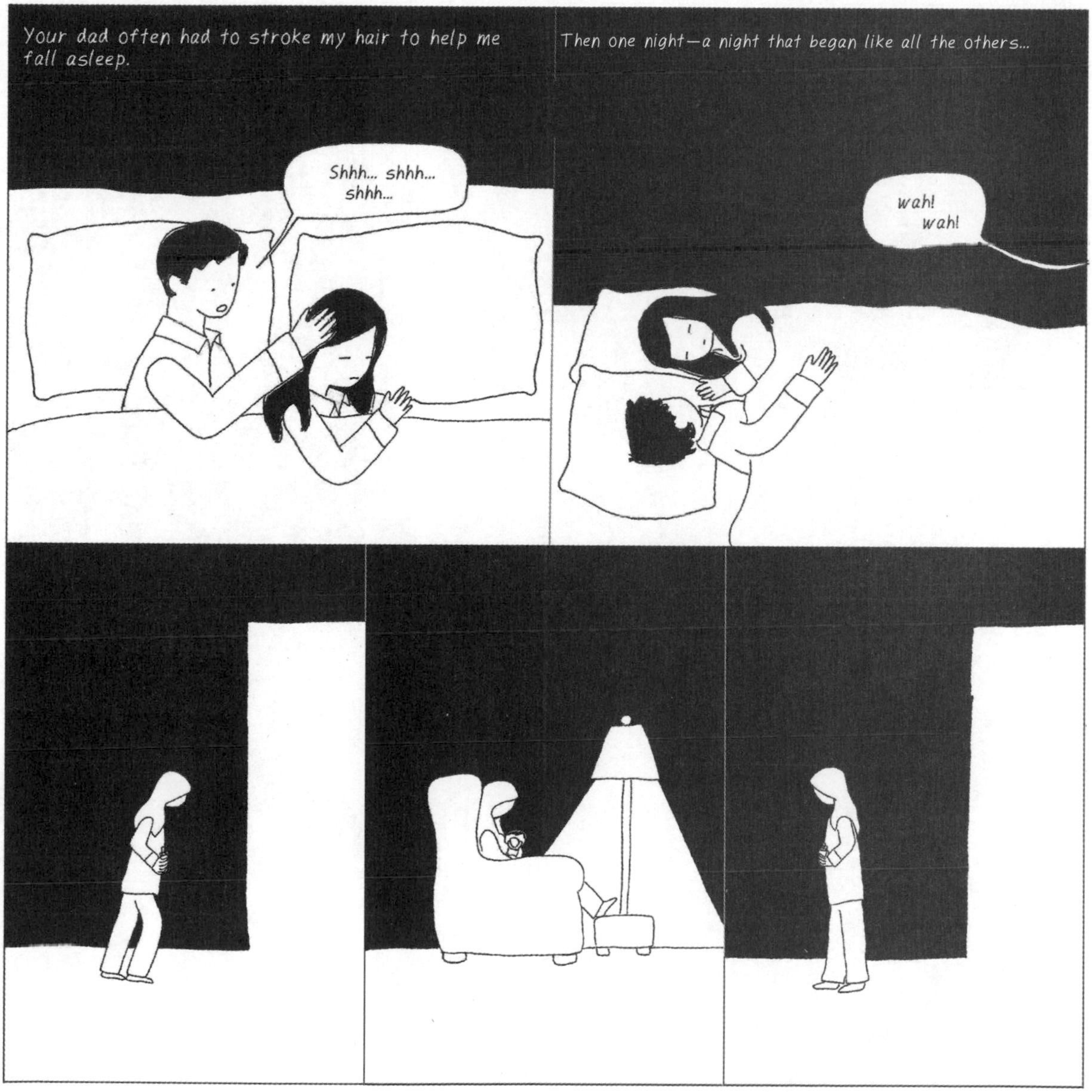
Your dad often had to stroke my hair to help me fall asleep.
Shhh... shhh... shhh...
Then one night—a night that began like all the others...
wah! wah!

It took me some time to fall back to sleep.
And when I finally drifted off...
wah! wah!
wah! wah!
wah! wah!

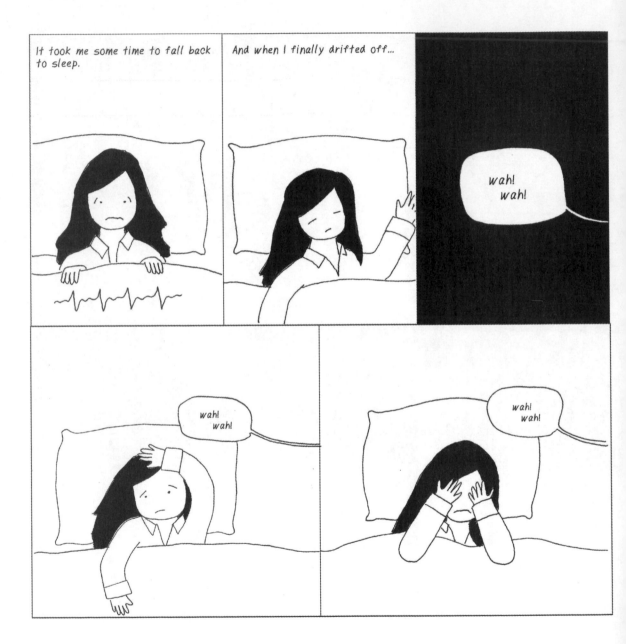

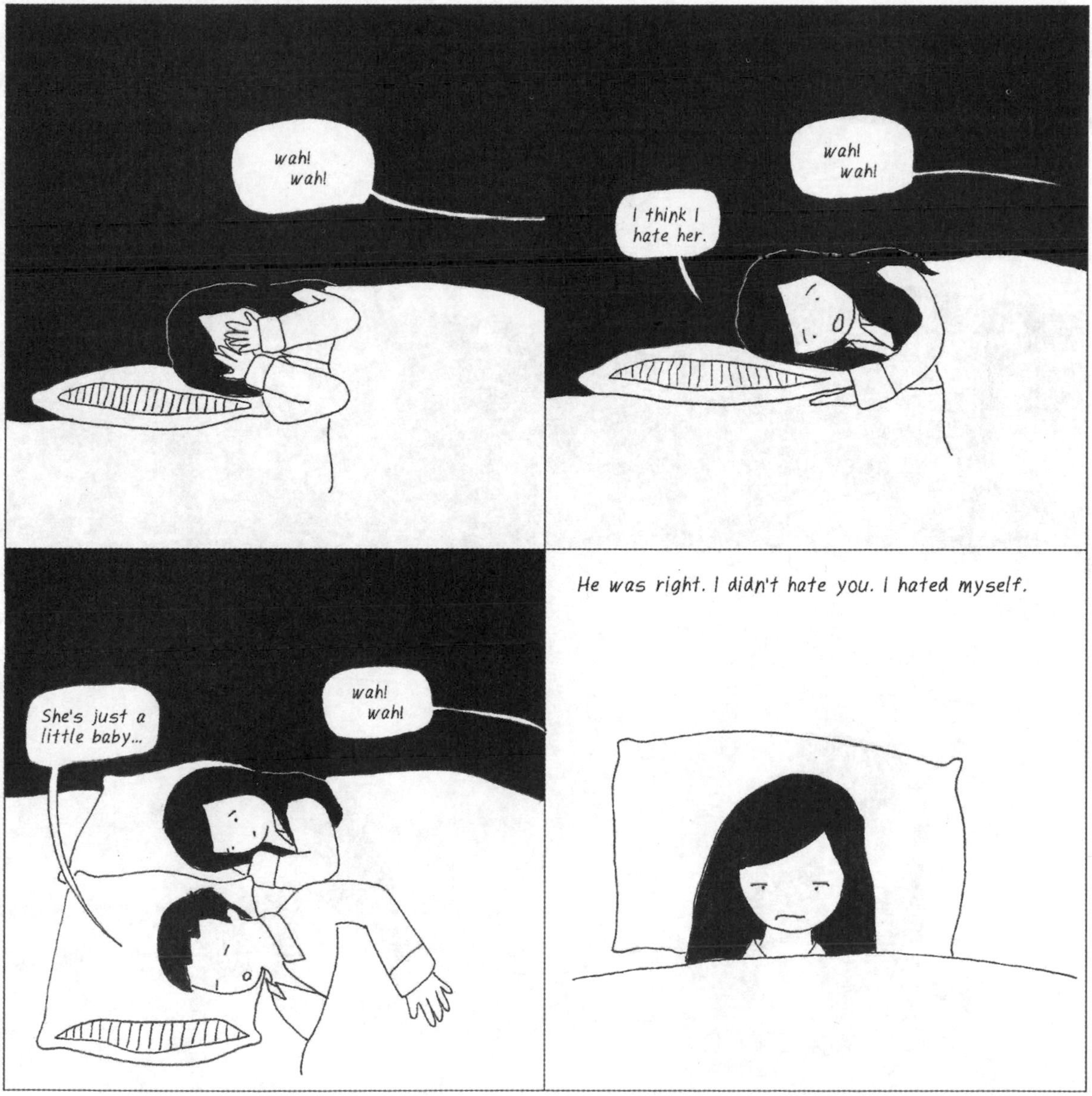
wah! wah!
wah! wah!
I think I hate her.
She's just a little baby...
wah! wah!
He was right. I didn't hate you. I hated myself.

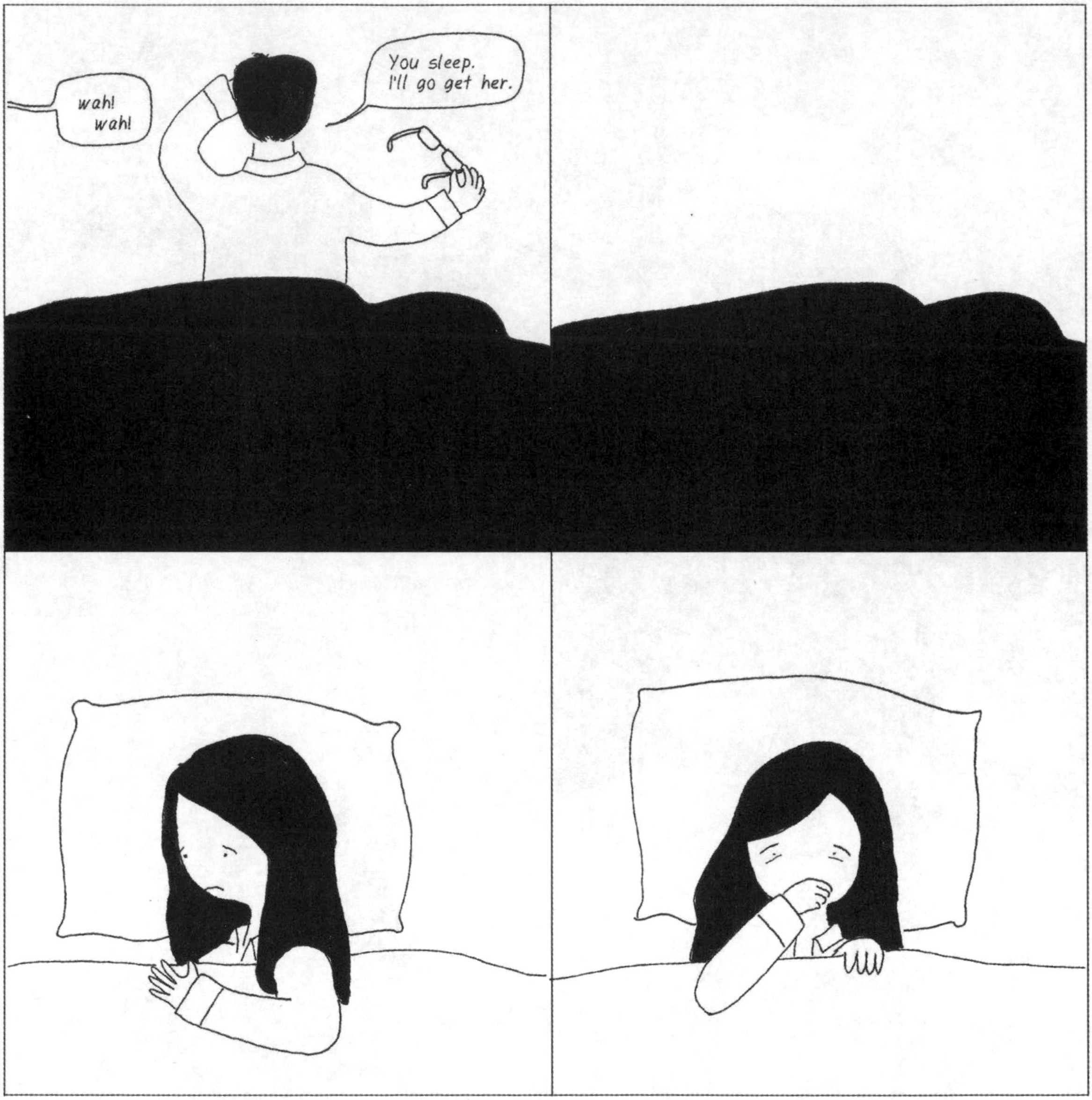
wah!
wah!
You sleep.
I'll go get her.

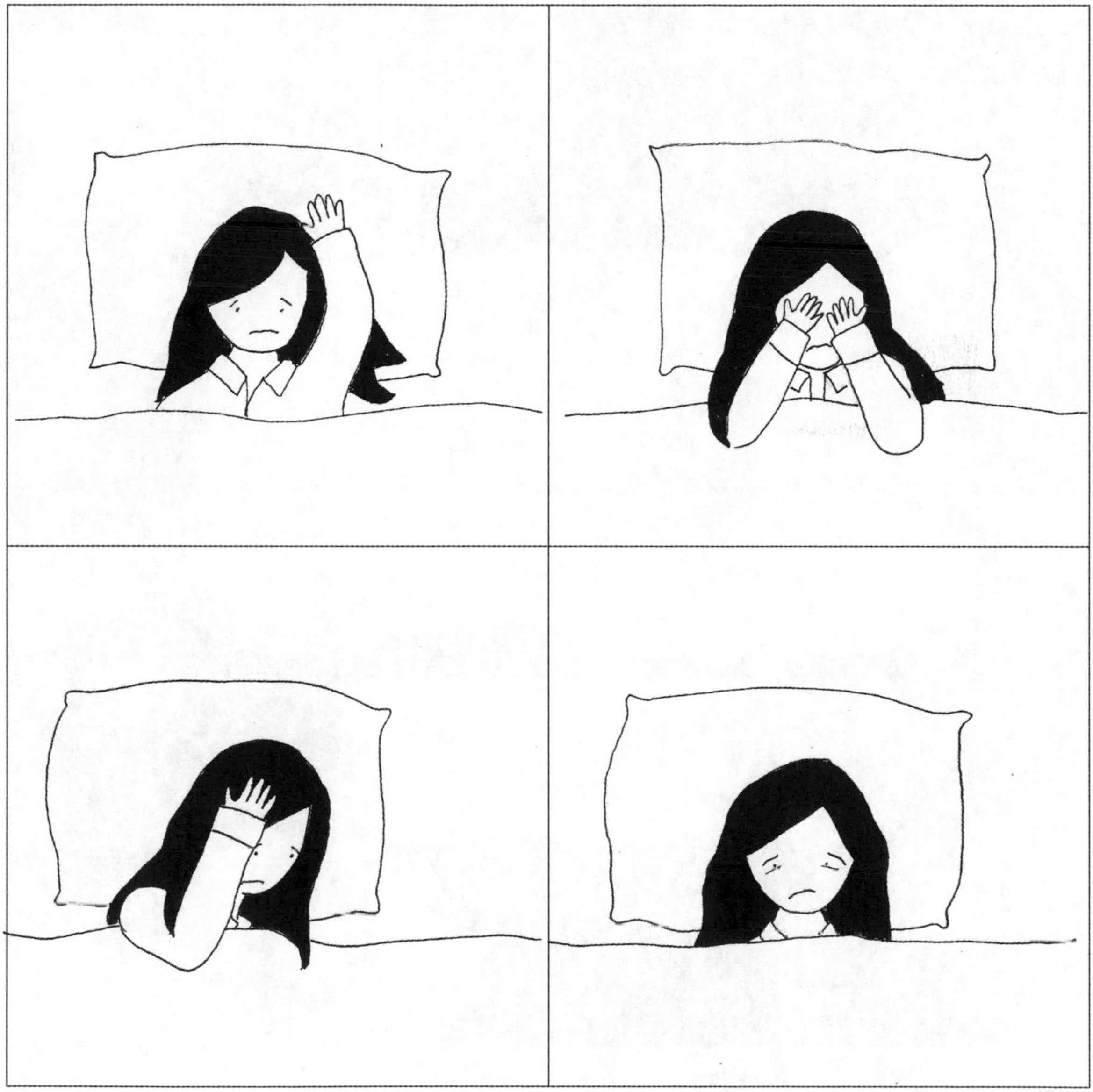

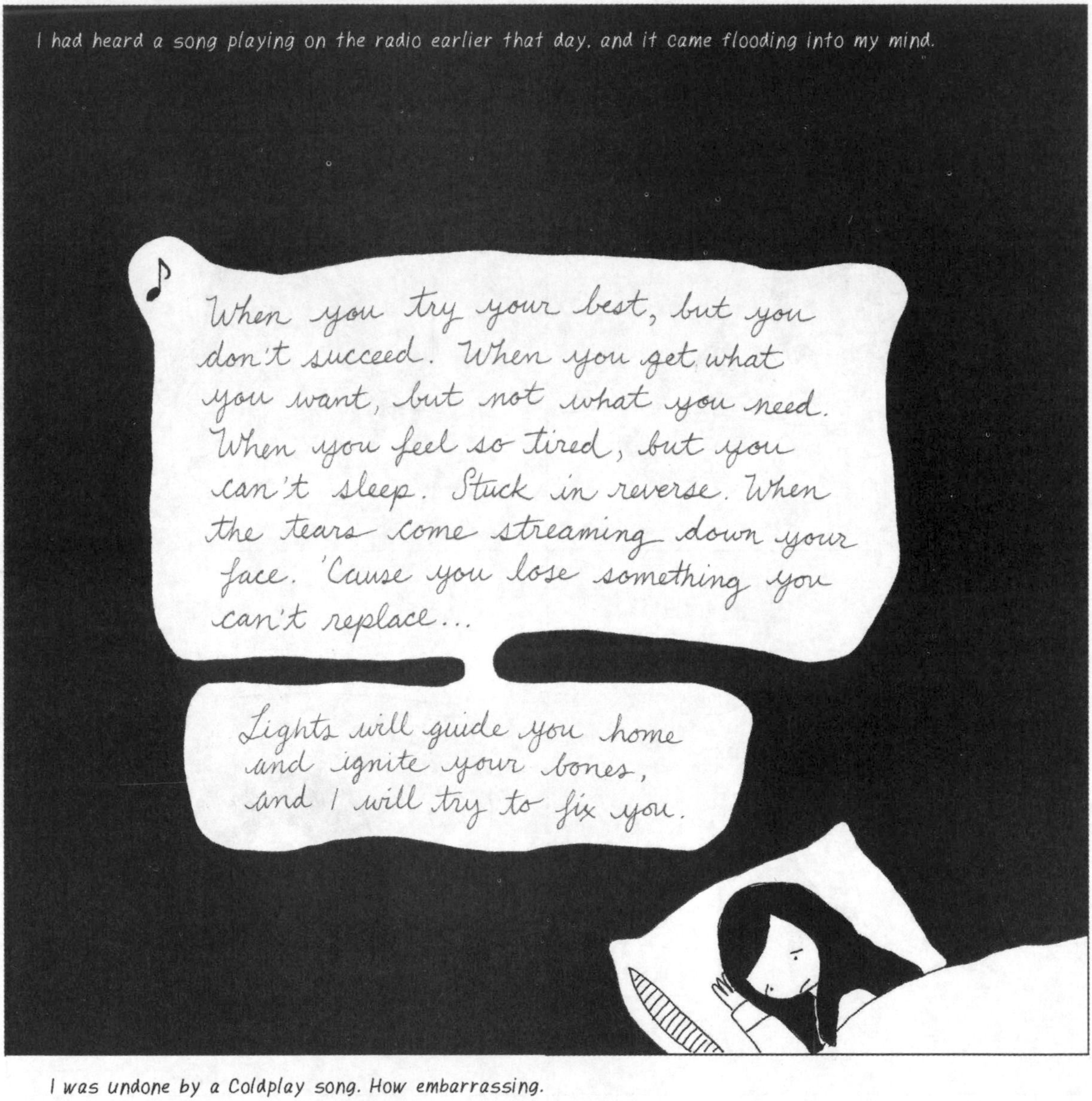
I had heard a song playing on the radio earlier that day, and it came flooding into my mind.
When you try your best, but you don't succeed. When you get what you want, but not what you need. When you feel so tired, but you can't sleep. Stuck in reverse. When the tears come streaming down your face. 'Cause you lose something you can't replace...
Lights will guide you home and ignite your bones, and I will try to fix you.

I was undone by a Coldplay song. How embarrassing.

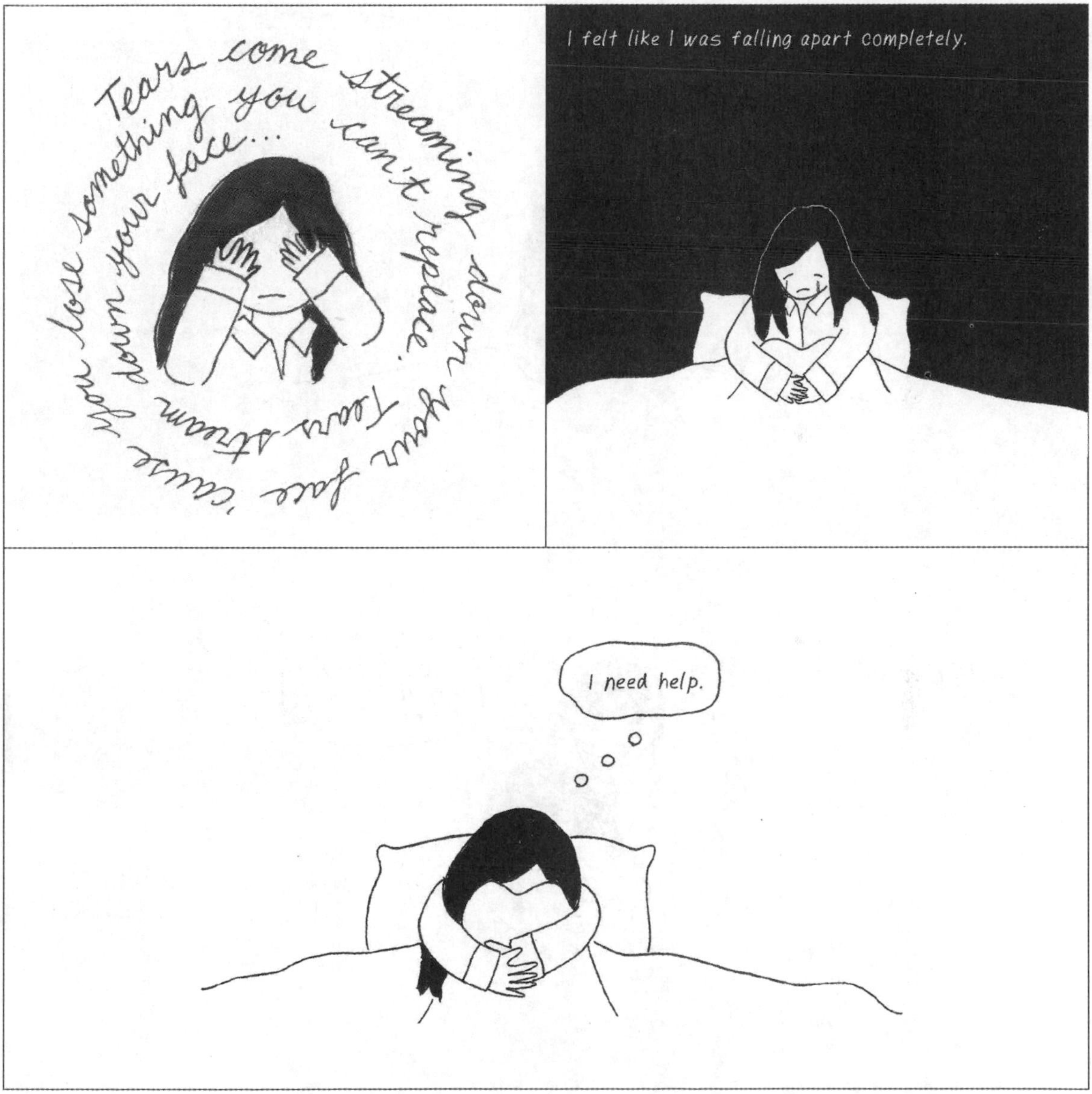
Tears come streaming down your face 'cause you lose something you can't replace. Tears stream down your face...
I felt like I was falling apart completely.
I need help.

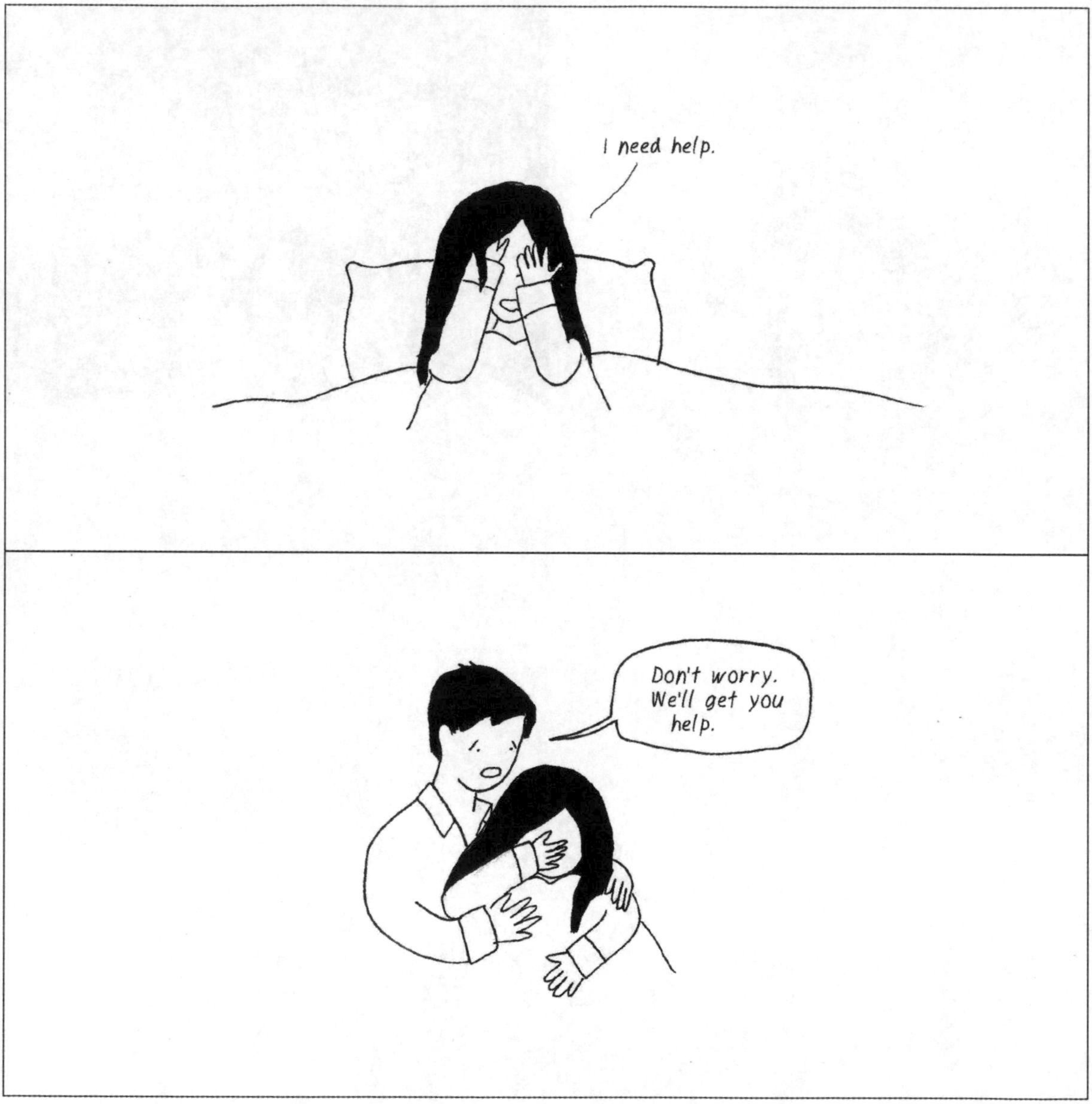
I need help.
Don't worry. We'll get you help.

The diagnosis was textbook, really...

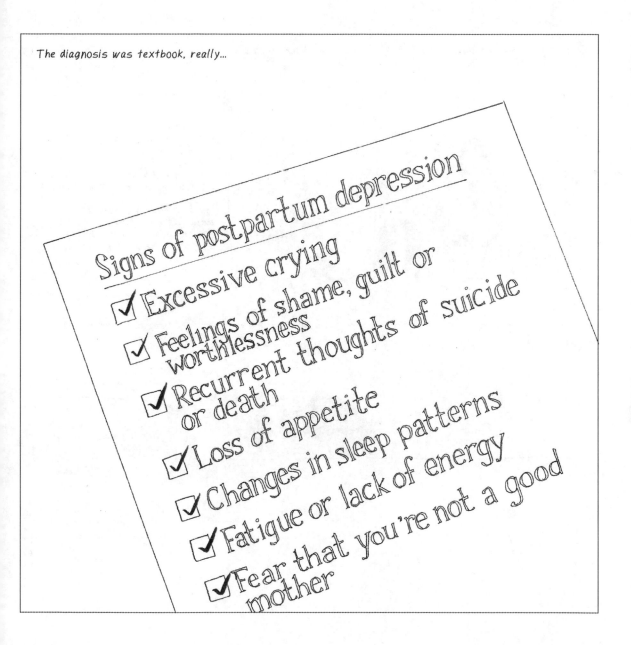

Signs of postpartum depression

☑ Excessive crying

☑ Feelings of shame, guilt or worthlessness

☑ Recurrent thoughts of suicide or death

☑ Loss of appetite

☑ Changes in sleep patterns

☑ Fatigue or lack of energy

☑ Fear that you're not a good mother

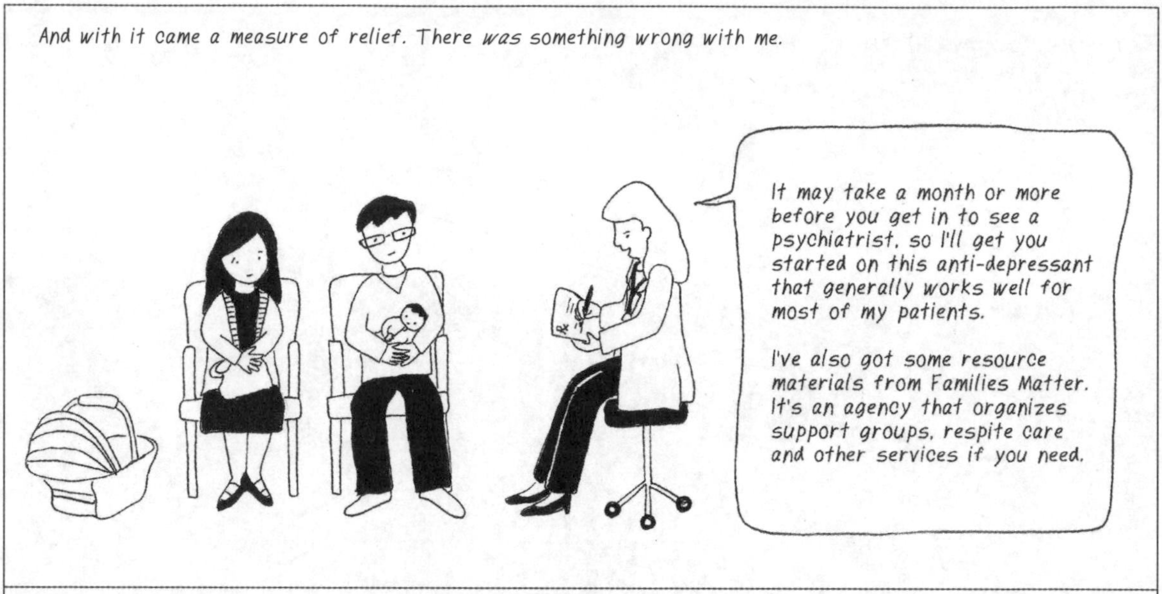
And with it came a measure of relief. There *was* something wrong with me.
It may take a month or more before you get in to see a psychiatrist, so I'll get you started on this anti-depressant that generally works well for most of my patients.
I've also got some resource materials from Families Matter. It's an agency that organizes support groups, respite care and other services if you need.

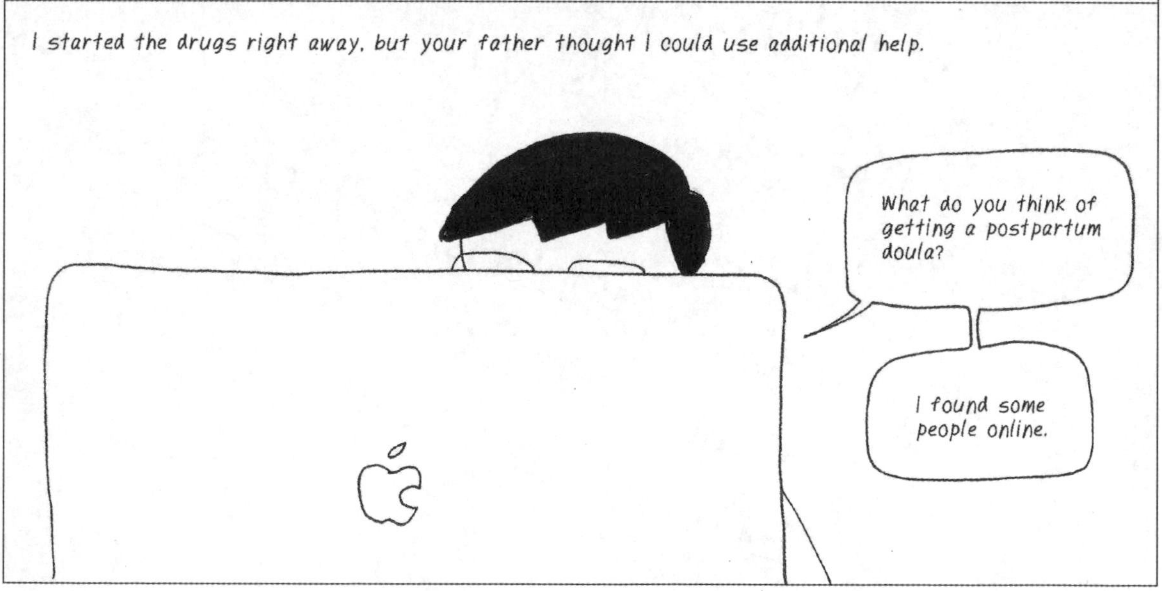
I started the drugs right away, but your father thought I could use additional help.
What do you think of getting a postpartum doula?
I found some people online.

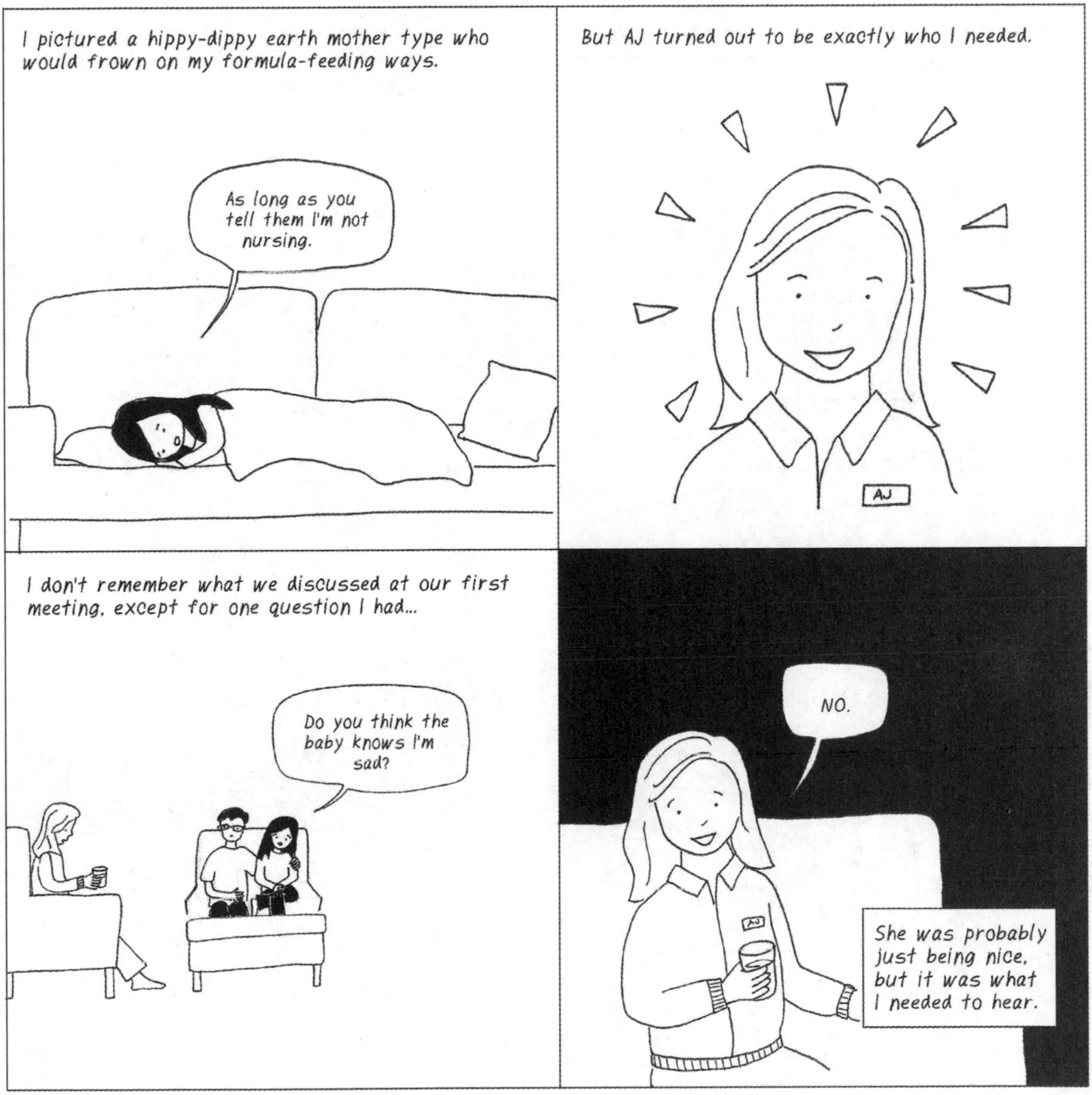
I pictured a hippy-dippy earth mother type who would frown on my formula-feeding ways.
As long as you tell them I'm not nursing.
But AJ turned out to be exactly who I needed.
AJ
I don't remember what we discussed at our first meeting, except for one question I had...
Do you think the baby knows I'm sad?
NO.
AJ
She was probably just being nice, but it was what I needed to hear.

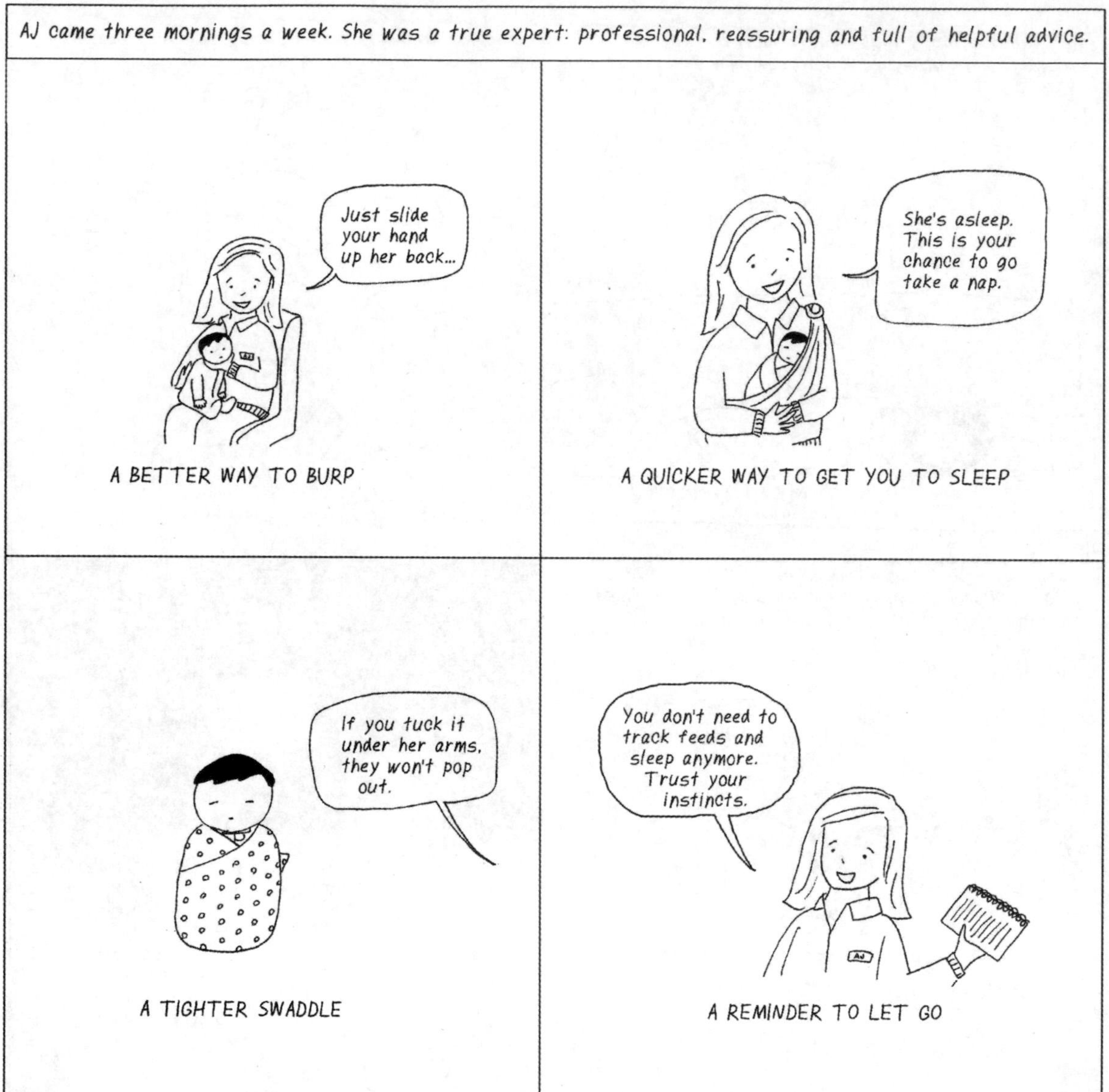
AJ came three mornings a week. She was a true expert: professional, reassuring and full of helpful advice.
Just slide your hand up her back...
A BETTER WAY TO BURP
She's asleep. This is your chance to go take a nap.
A QUICKER WAY TO GET YOU TO SLEEP
If you tuck it under her arms, they won't pop out.
A TIGHTER SWADDLE
You don't need to track feeds and sleep anymore. Trust your instincts.
AJ
A REMINDER TO LET GO

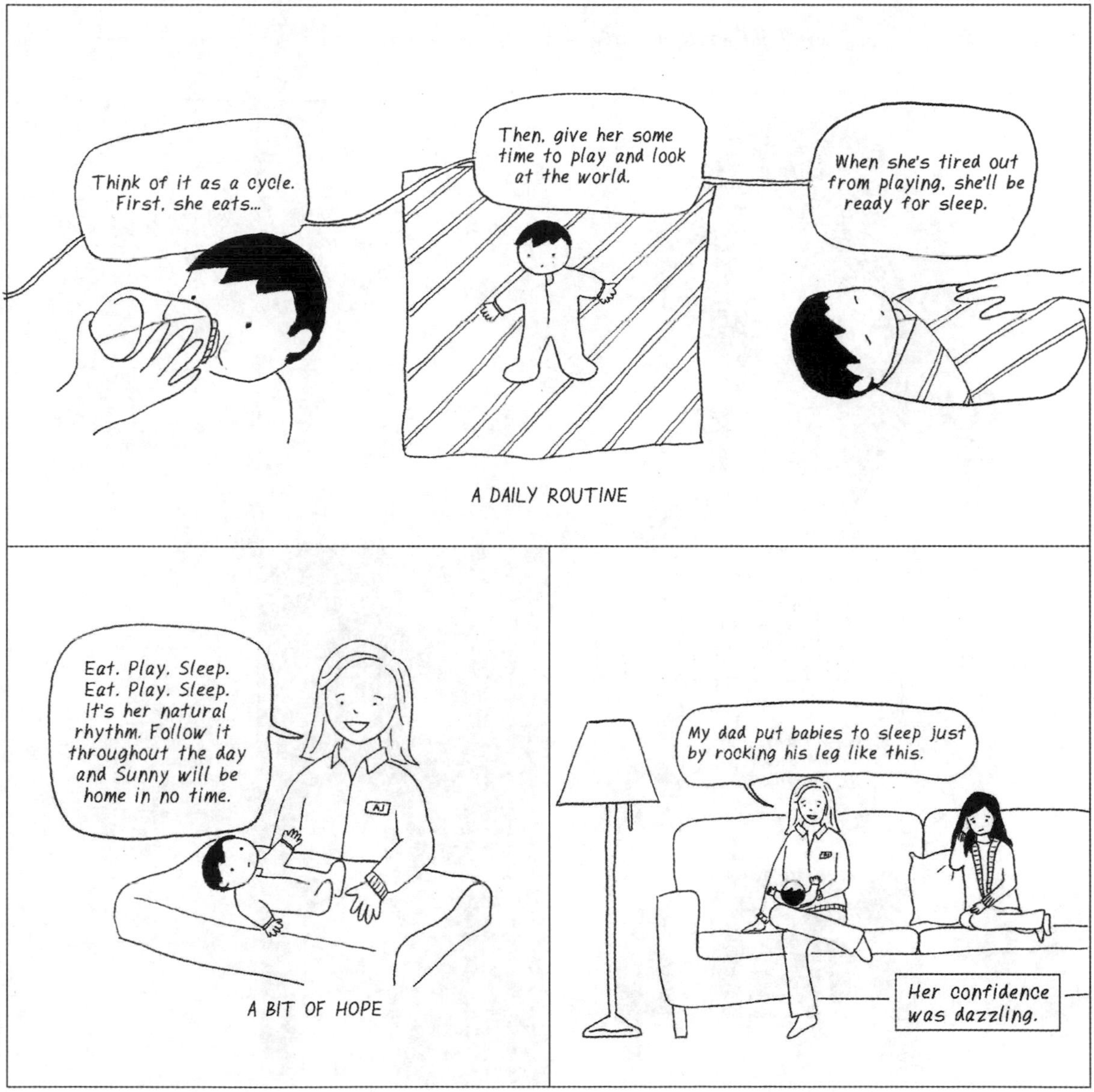
Think of it as a cycle. First, she eats...
Then, give her some time to play and look at the world.
When she's tired out from playing, she'll be ready for sleep.
A DAILY ROUTINE
Eat. Play. Sleep. Eat. Play. Sleep. It's her natural rhythm. Follow it throughout the day and Sunny will be home in no time.
AJ
A BIT OF HOPE
My dad put babies to sleep just by rocking his leg like this.
Her confidence was dazzling.

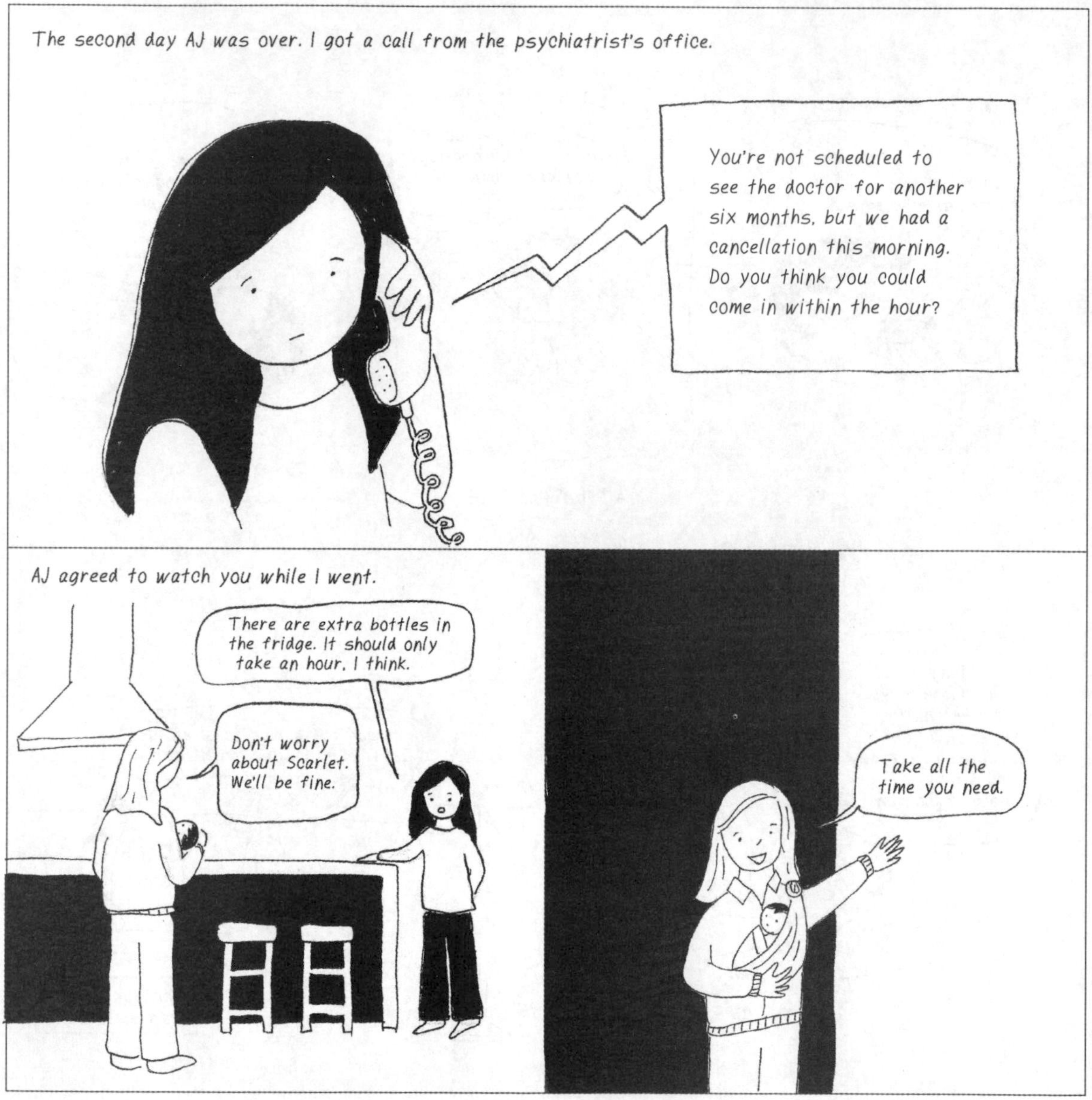

The second day AJ was over. I got a call from the psychiatrist's office.
You're not scheduled to see the doctor for another six months, but we had a cancellation this morning. Do you think you could come in within the hour?
AJ agreed to watch you while I went.
There are extra bottles in the fridge. It should only take an hour, I think.
Don't worry about Scarlet. We'll be fine.
Take all the time you need.

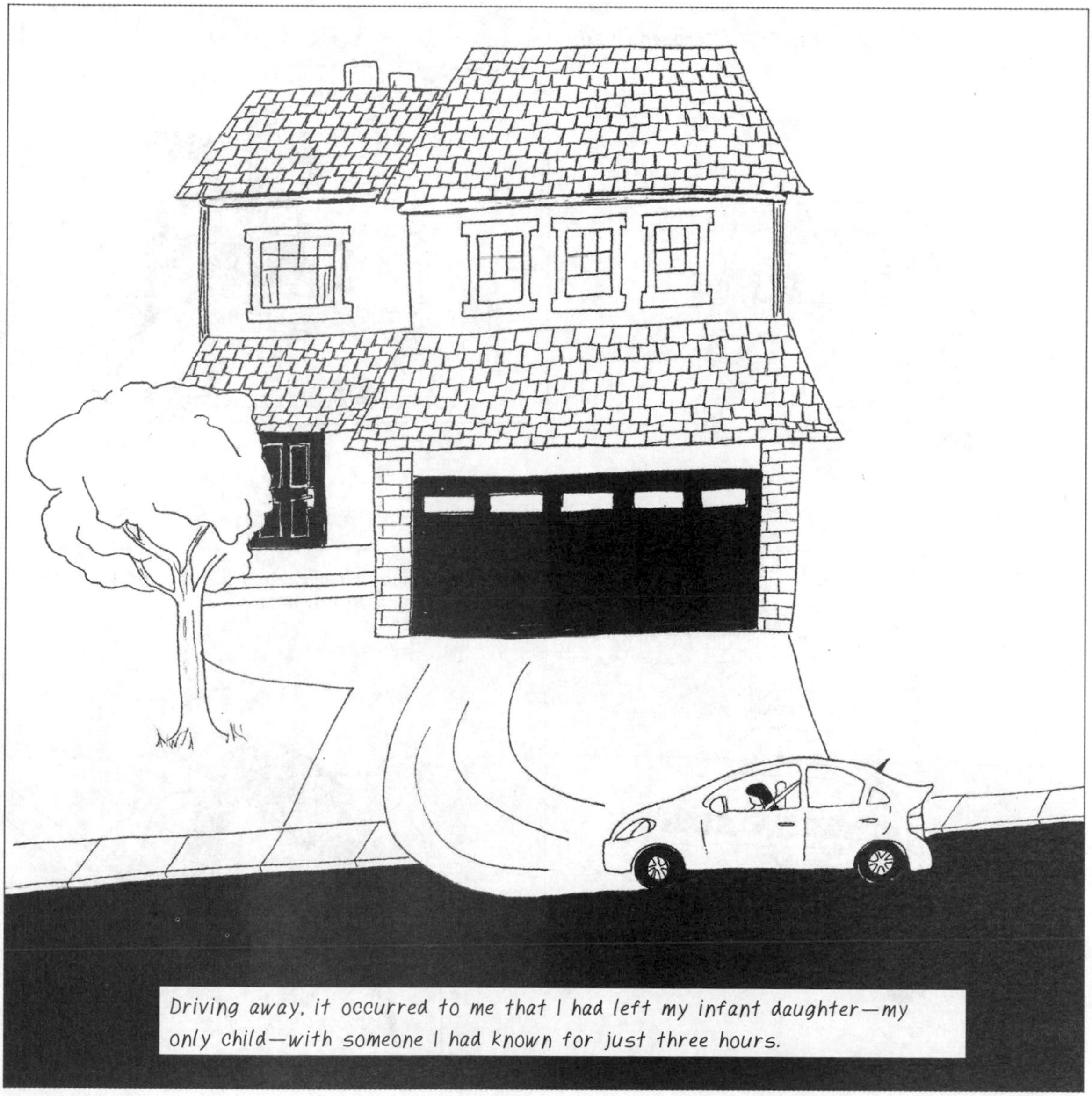
Driving away, it occurred to me that I had left my infant daughter—my only child—with someone I had known for just three hours.

I felt bad for a moment. Again, I had chosen myself over you.

But sometimes you have to take care of yourself before you can do anything else.

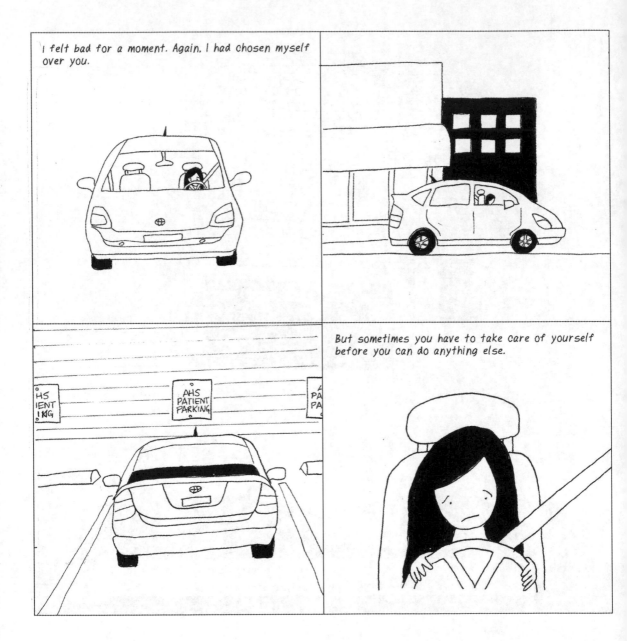

As they like to remind us on airplanes...

1
How can I be so selfish?
2
I should be thinking of her.
3
A good mother sacrifices herself...
4
So she can put her child first.

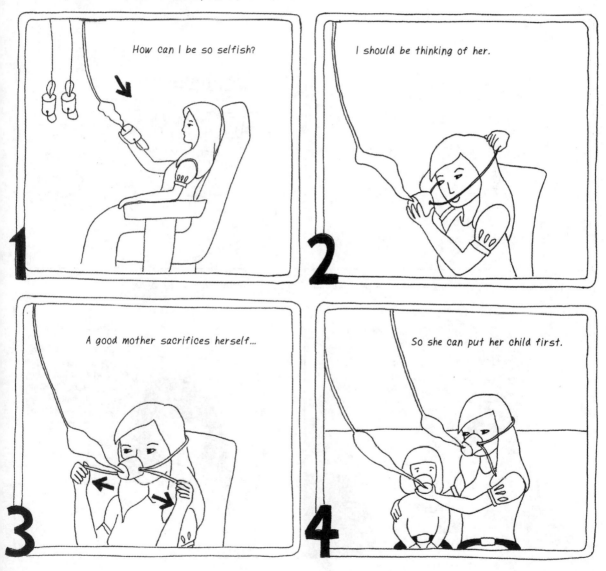

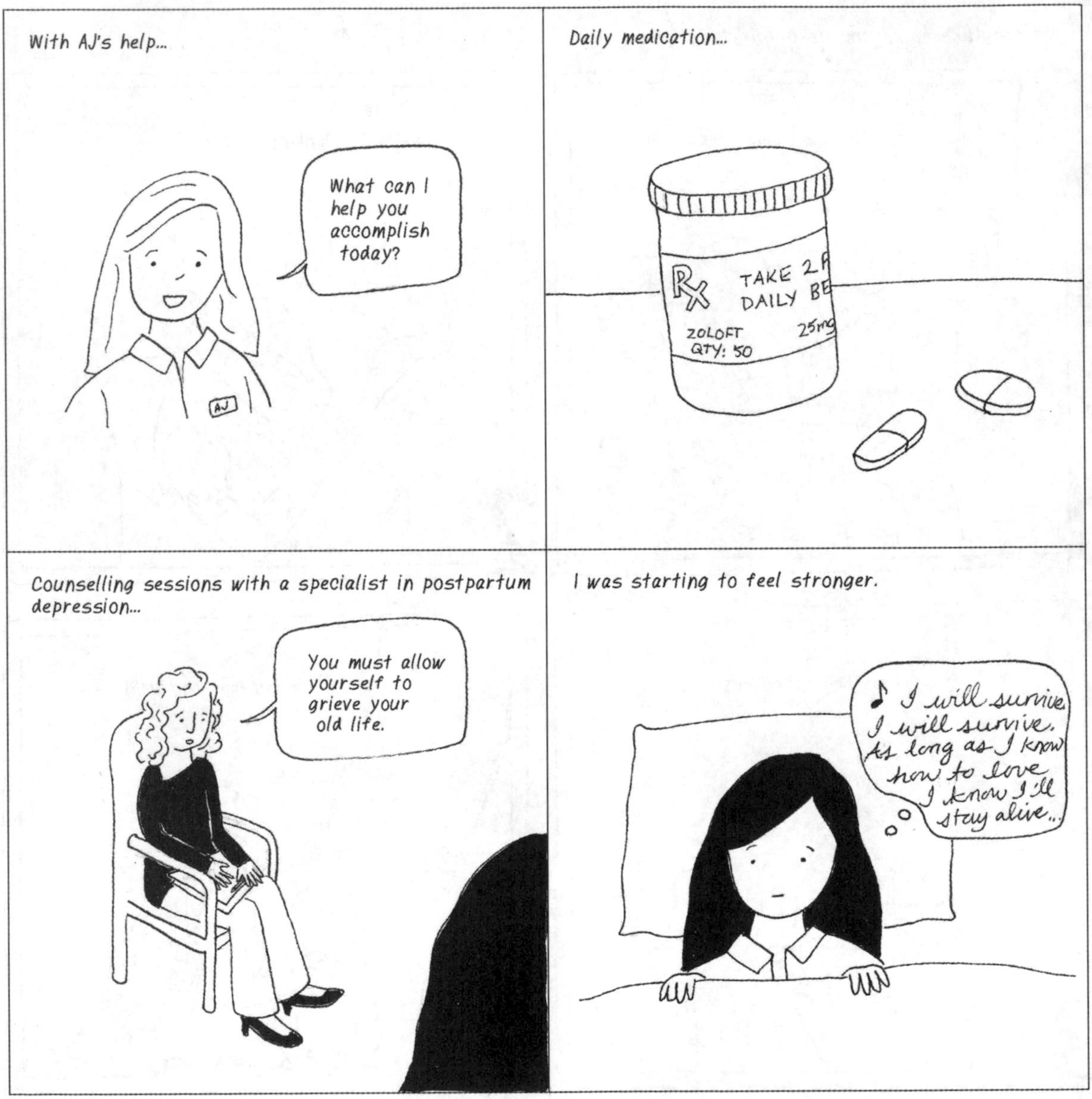
With AJ's help...
What can I help you accomplish today?
AJ
Daily medication...
Rx
TAKE 2
DAILY
ZOLOFT
25mg
QTY: 50
Counselling sessions with a specialist in postpartum depression...
You must allow yourself to grieve your old life.
I was starting to feel stronger.
♪ I will survive. I will survive. As long as I know how to love I know I'll stay alive...

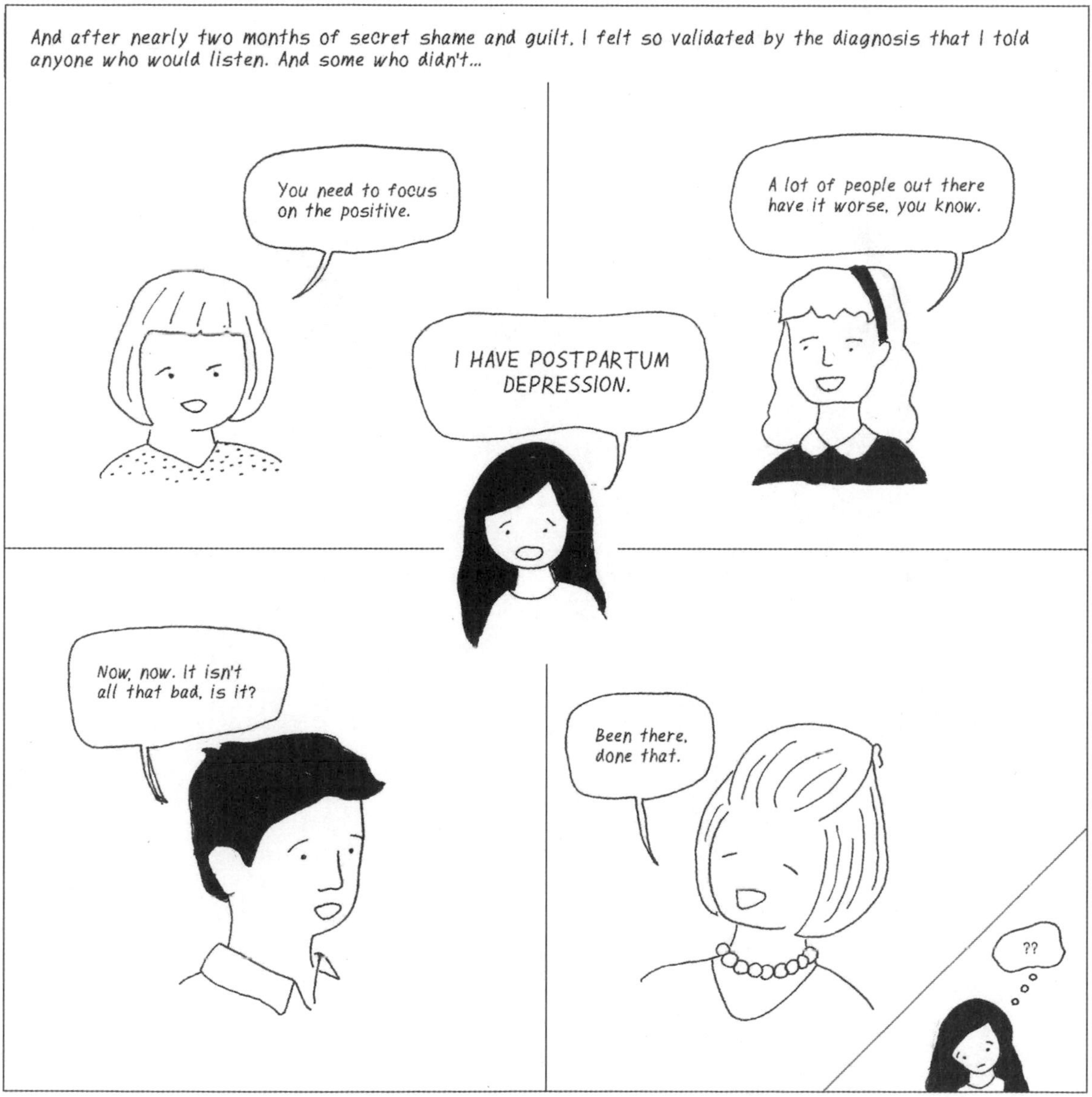
And after nearly two months of secret shame and guilt, I felt so validated by the diagnosis that I told anyone who would listen. And some who didn't...
I HAVE POSTPARTUM DEPRESSION.
You need to focus on the positive.
A lot of people out there have it worse, you know.
Now, now. It isn't all that bad, is it?
Been there, done that.
??

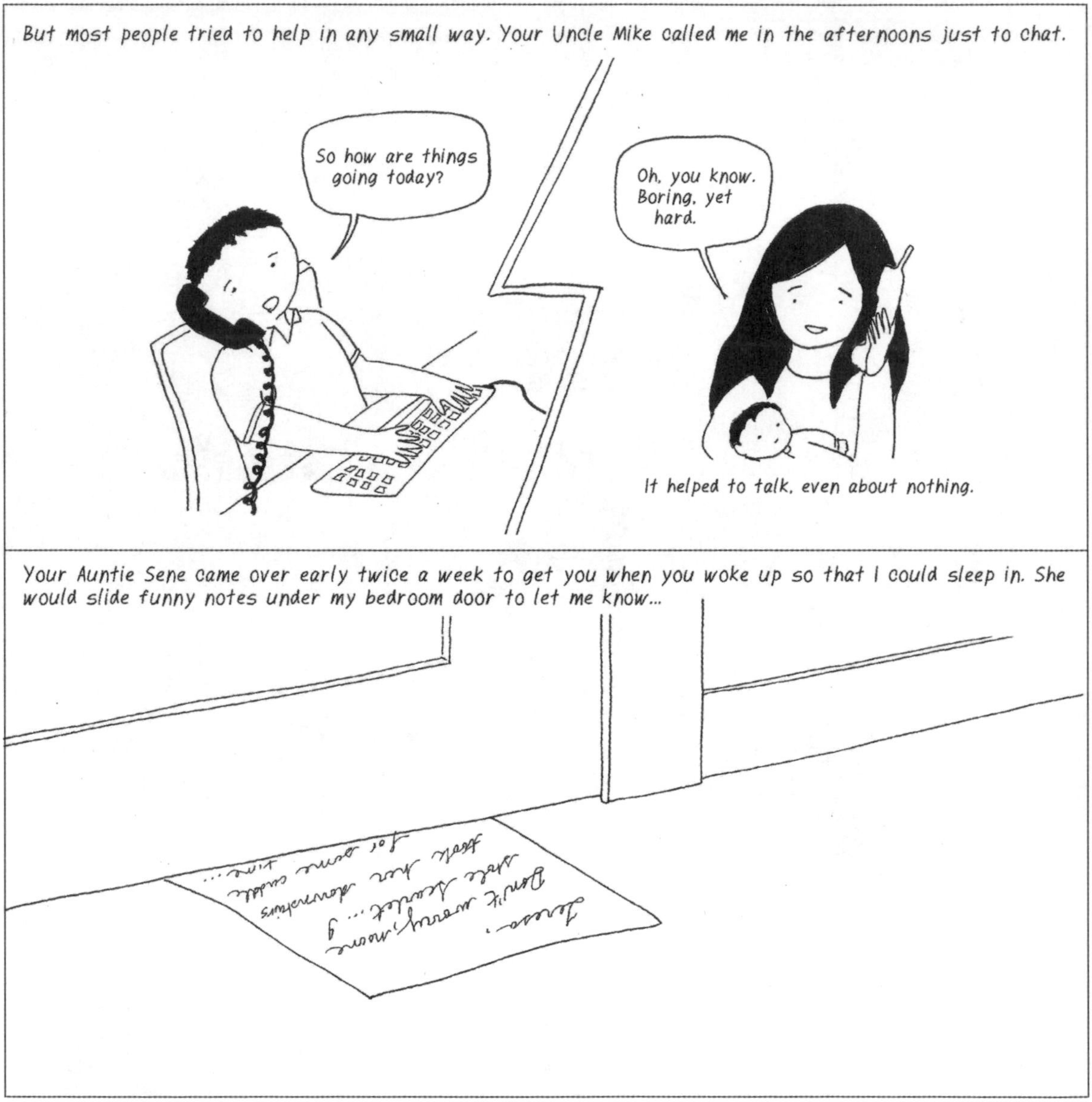
But most people tried to help in any small way. Your Uncle Mike called me in the afternoons just to chat.
So how are things going today?
Oh, you know. Boring, yet hard.
It helped to talk, even about nothing.
Your Auntie Sene came over early twice a week to get you when you woke up so that I could sleep in. She would slide funny notes under my bedroom door to let me know...

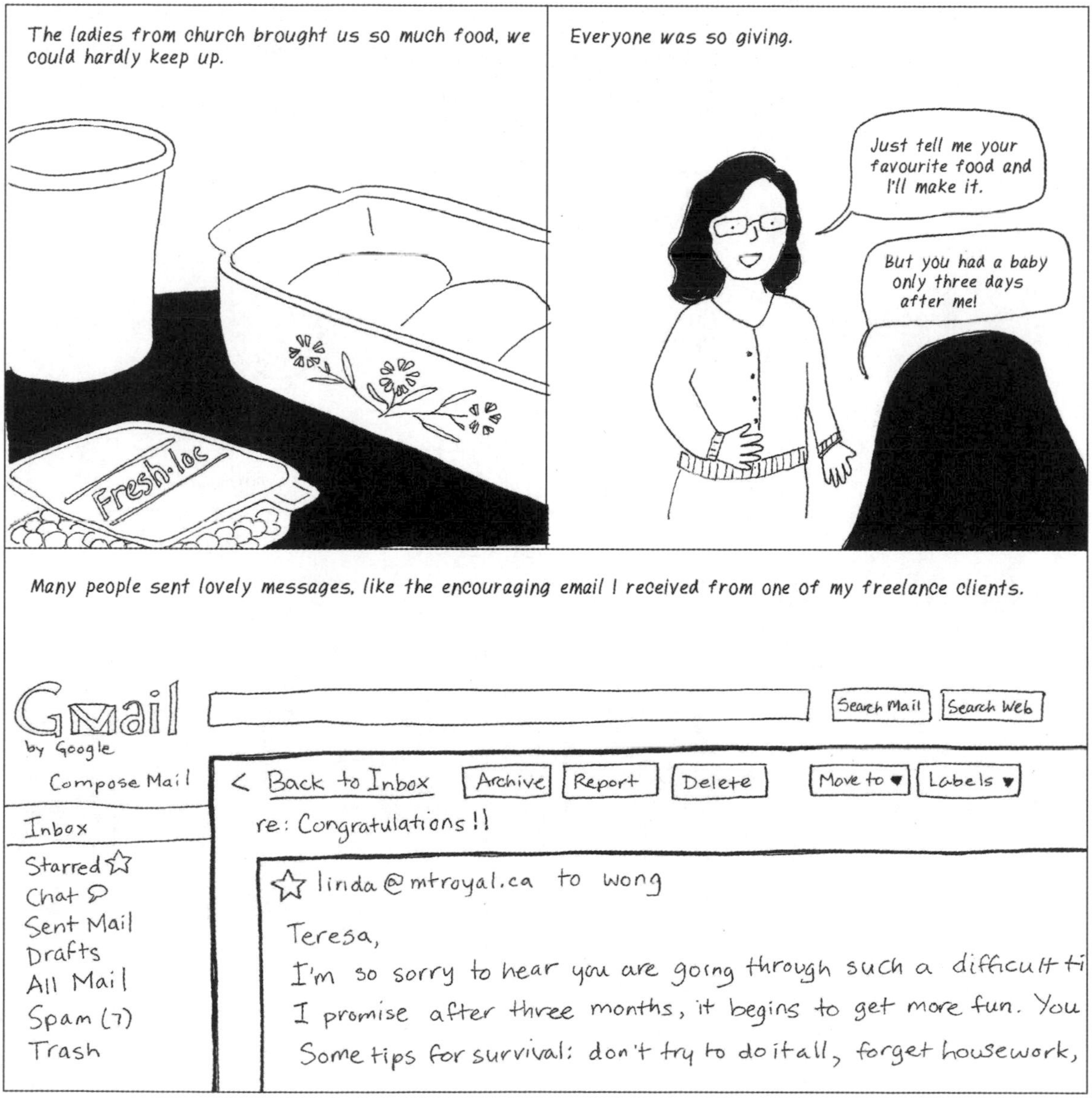
The ladies from church brought us so much food, we could hardly keep up.
Fresh·loc
Everyone was so giving.
Just tell me your favourite food and I'll make it.
But you had a baby only three days after me!
Many people sent lovely messages, like the encouraging email I received from one of my freelance clients.
Gmail
by Google
Search Mail
Search Web
Compose Mail
< Back to Inbox
Archive
Report
Delete
Move to ▾
Labels ▾
Inbox
re: Congratulations!!
Starred
Chat
Sent Mail
Drafts
All Mail
Spam (7)
Trash
linda@mtroyal.ca to wong
Teresa,
I'm so sorry to hear you are going through such a difficult ti
I promise after three months, it begins to get more fun. You
Some tips for survival: don't try to do it all, forget housework,

MOMS WHO HAD POSTPARTUM

* NOT ONE OF THEM FAINT OF HEART *

As I shared my struggles, others began to share theirs with me, making me feel like part of a quiet sisterhood.

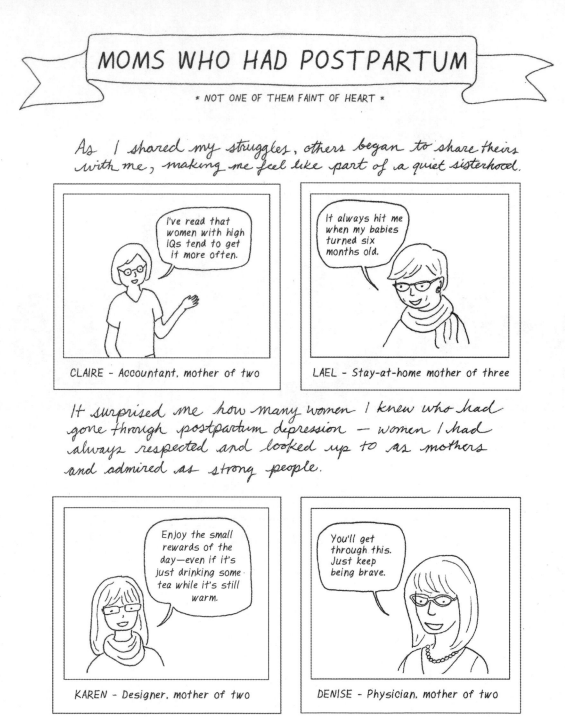

> I've read that women with high IQs tend to get it more often.

CLAIRE - Accountant, mother of two

> It always hit me when my babies turned six months old.

LAEL - Stay-at-home mother of three

It surprised me how many women I knew who had gone through postpartum depression — women I had always respected and looked up to as mothers and admired as strong people.

> Enjoy the small rewards of the day—even if it's just drinking some tea while it's still warm.

KAREN - Designer, mother of two

> You'll get through this. Just keep being brave.

DENISE - Physician, mother of two

I also noticed that they all wore glasses, but that is probably irrelevant.

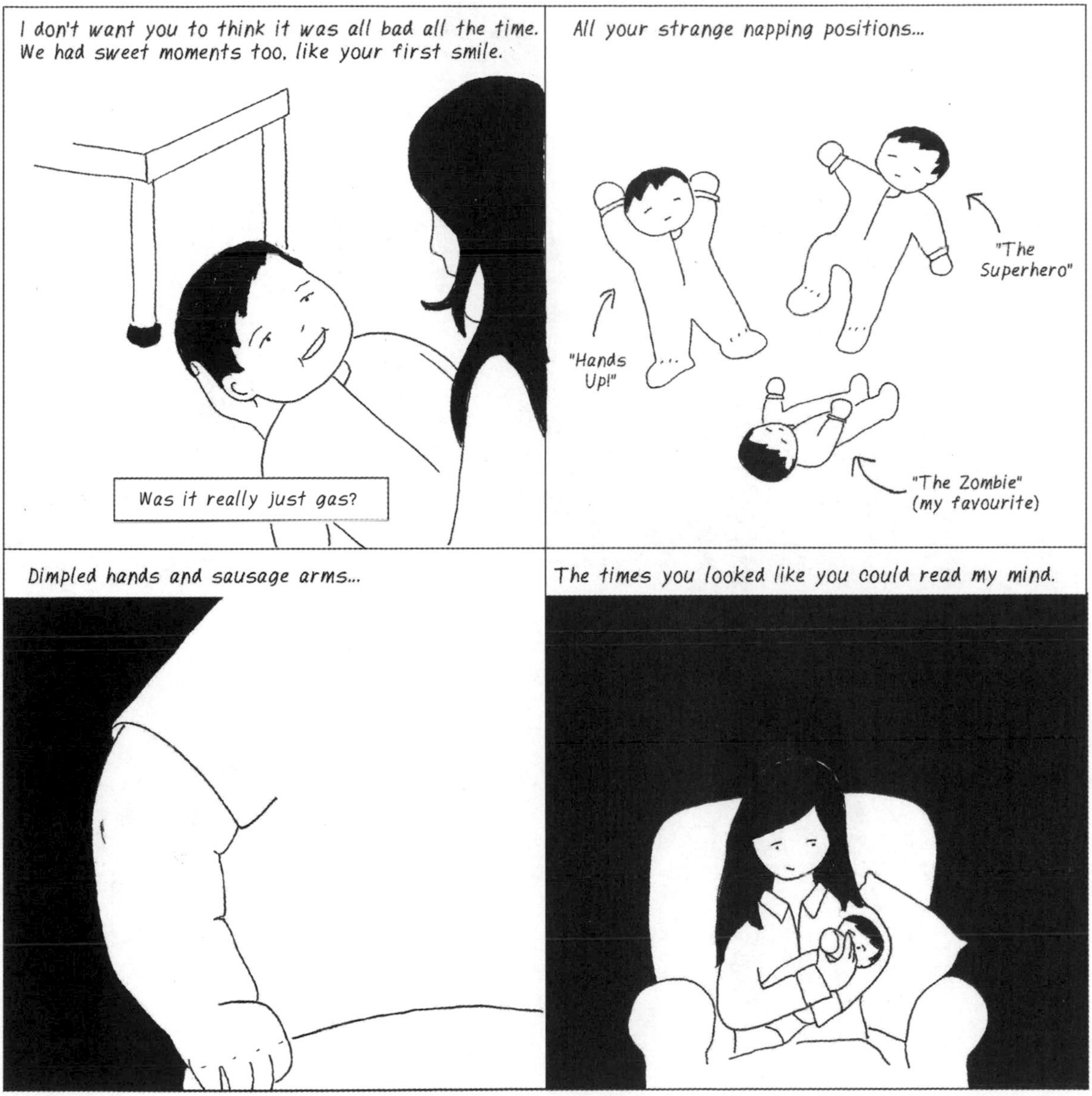
I don't want you to think it was all bad all the time. We had sweet moments too, like your first smile.
Was it really just gas?
All your strange napping positions...
"Hands Up!"
"The Superhero"
"The Zombie" (my favourite)
Dimpled hands and sausage arms...
The times you looked like you could read my mind.

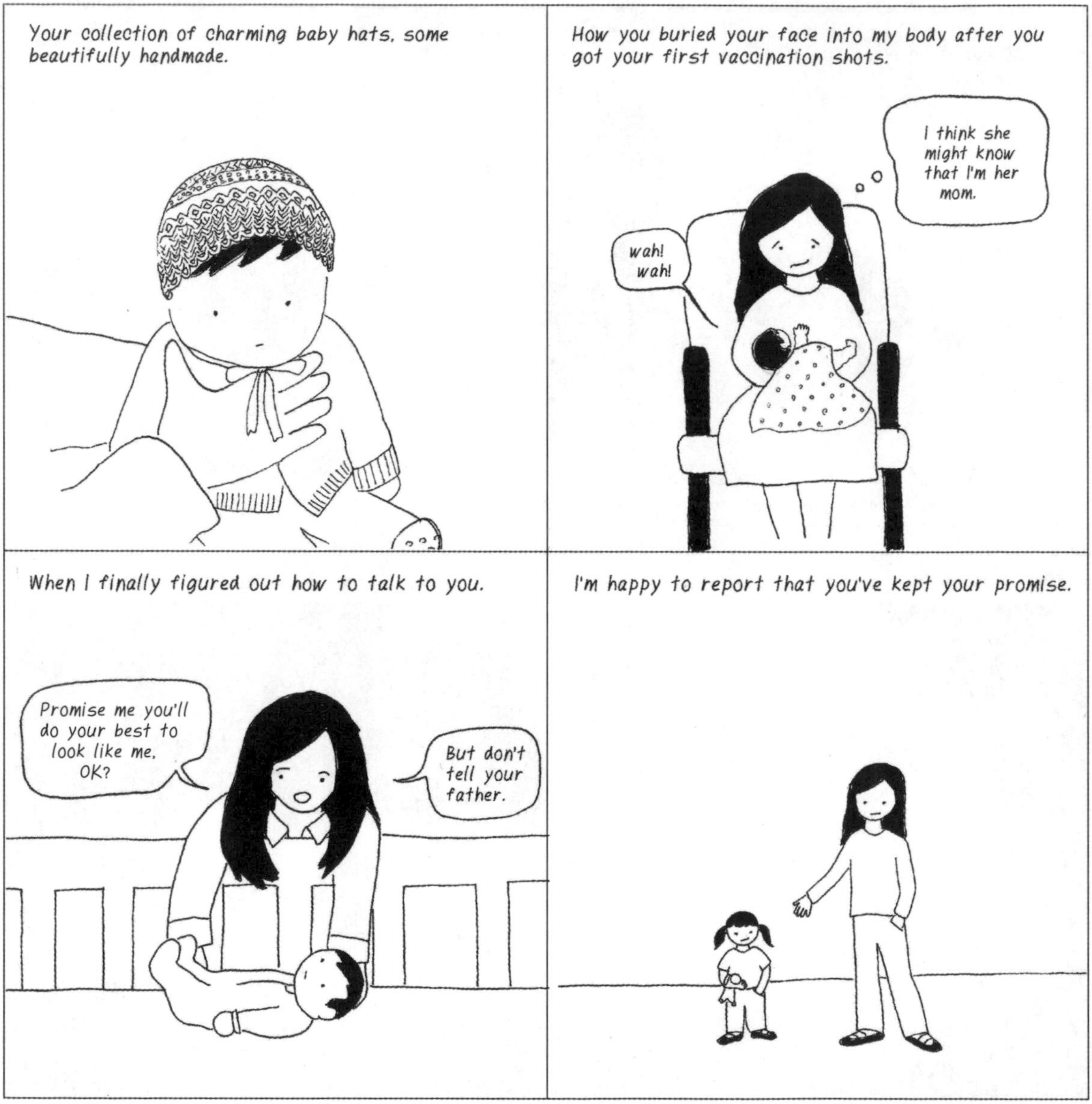
Your collection of charming baby hats, some beautifully handmade.
How you buried your face into my body after you got your first vaccination shots.
wah! wah!
I think she might know that I'm her mom.
When I finally figured out how to talk to you.
Promise me you'll do your best to look like me, OK?
But don't tell your father.
I'm happy to report that you've kept your promise.

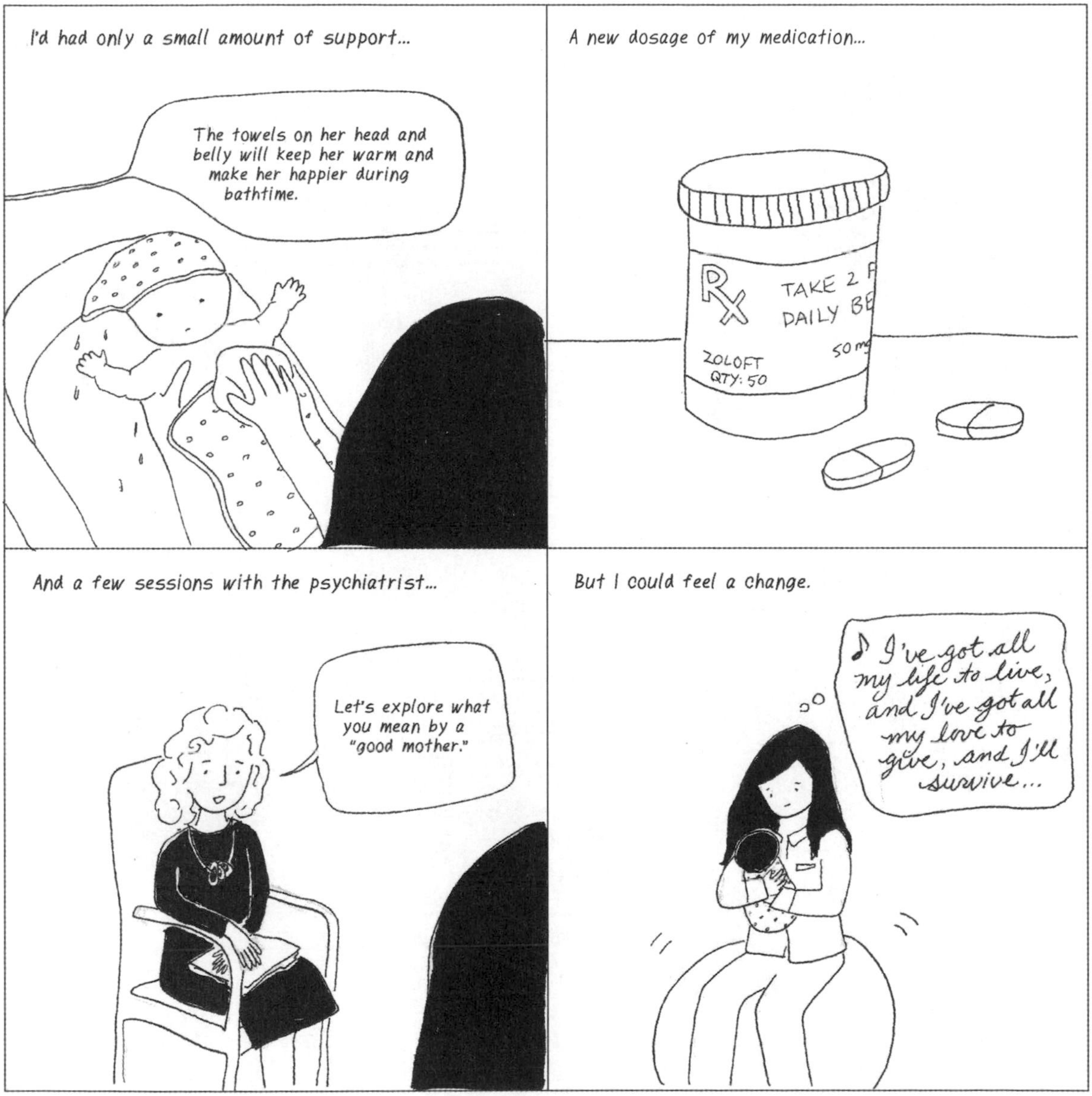
I'd had only a small amount of support...
The towels on her head and belly will keep her warm and make her happier during bathtime.
A new dosage of my medication...
RX TAKE 2 DAILY BE
ZOLOFT QTY: 50
And a few sessions with the psychiatrist...
Let's explore what you mean by a "good mother."
But I could feel a change.
♪ I've got all my life to live, and I've got all my love to give, and I'll survive...

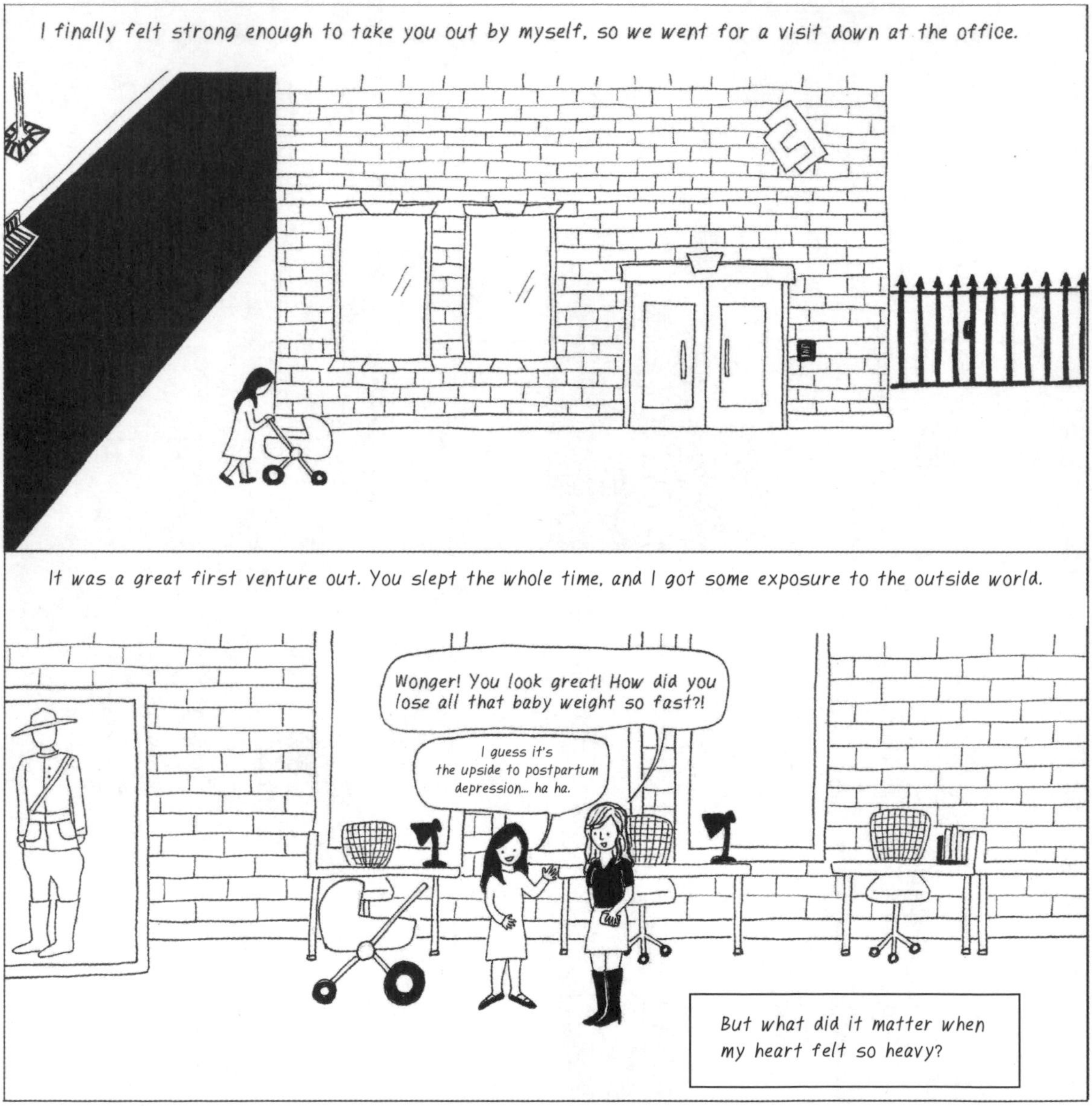
I finally felt strong enough to take you out by myself, so we went for a visit down at the office.
It was a great first venture out. You slept the whole time, and I got some exposure to the outside world.
Wonger! You look great! How did you lose all that baby weight so fast?!
I guess it's the upside to postpartum depression... ha ha.
But what did it matter when my heart felt so heavy?

For our next outing, I took you to see *Real Life*, the Ron Mueck exhibit at the Glenbow Museum.

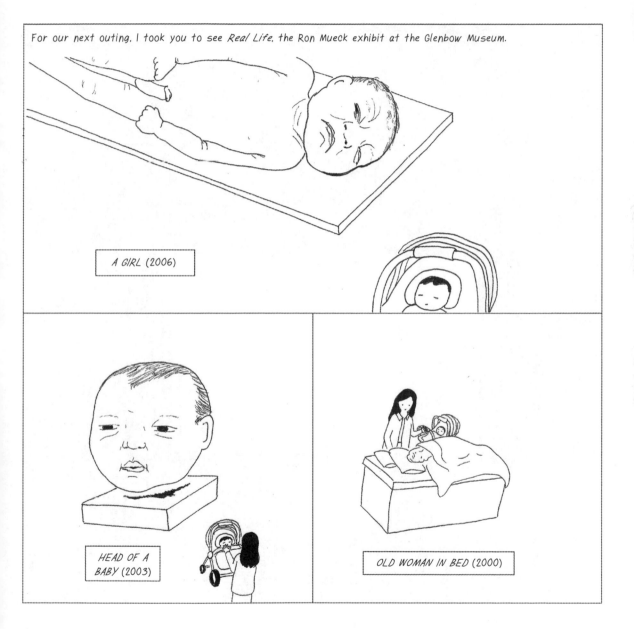

A GIRL (2006)

HEAD OF A
BABY (2003)

OLD WOMAN IN BED (2000)

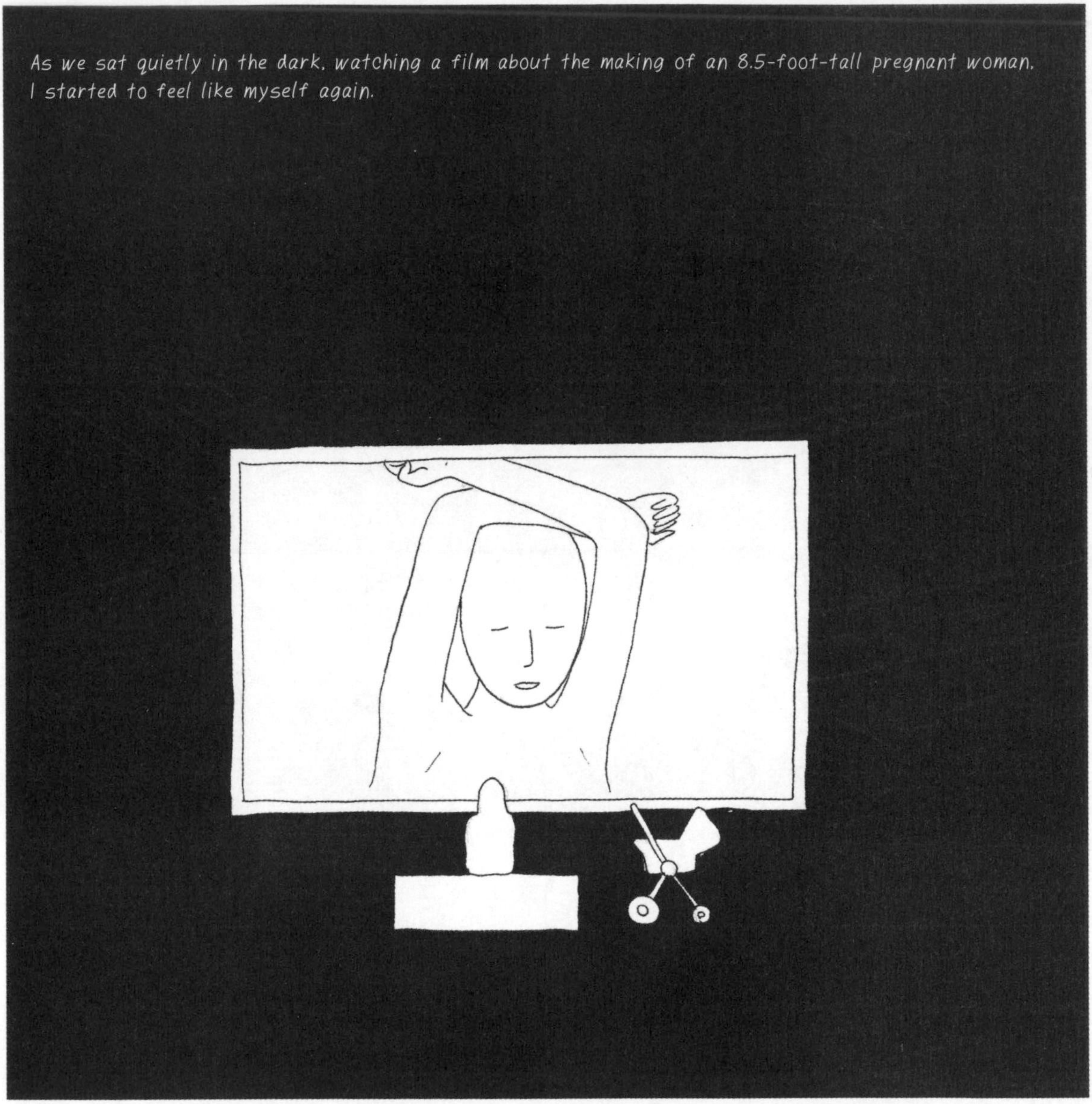
As we sat quietly in the dark, watching a film about the making of an 8.5-foot-tall pregnant woman, I started to feel like myself again.

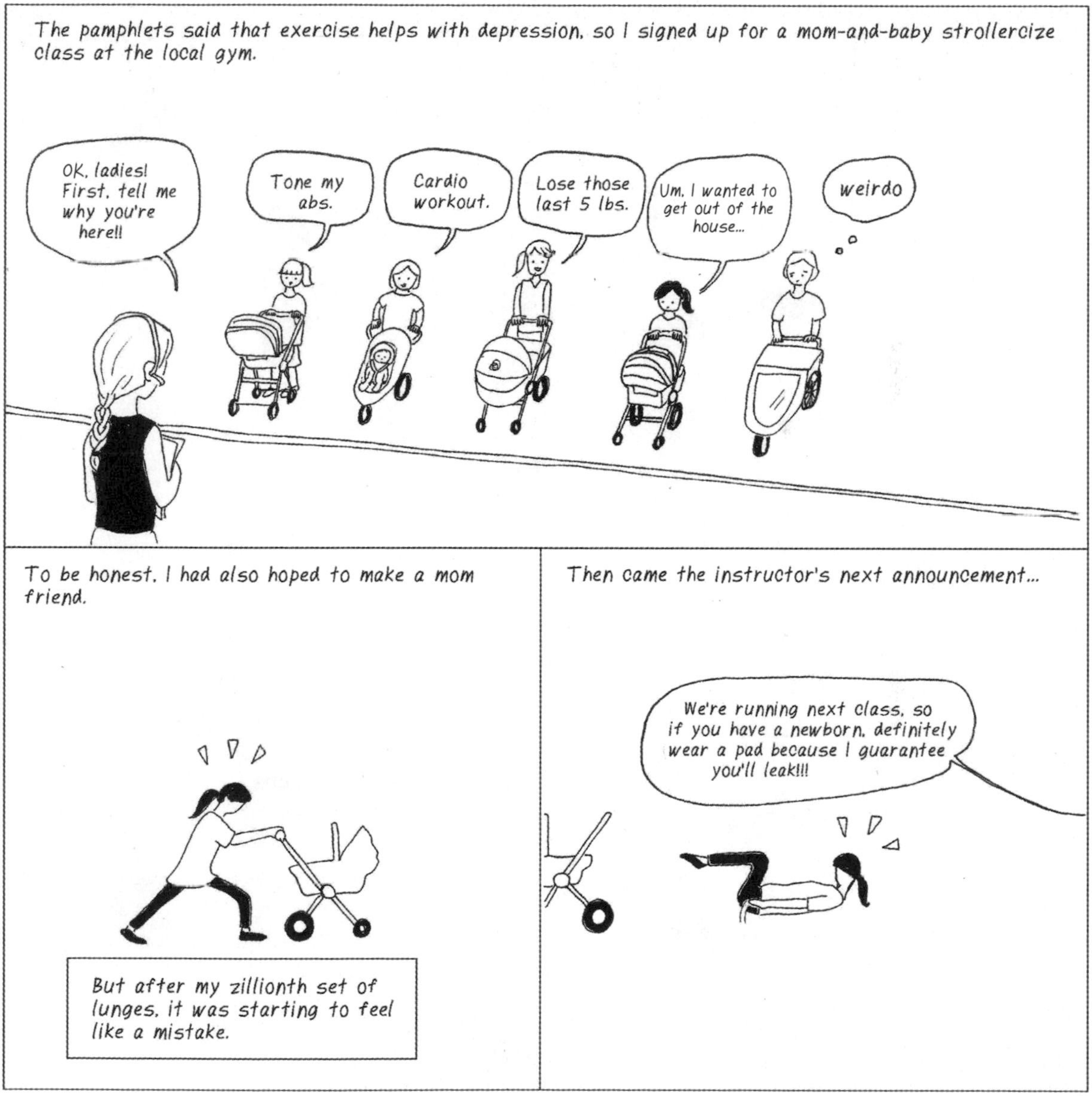
The pamphlets said that exercise helps with depression, so I signed up for a mom-and-baby strollercize class at the local gym.
OK, ladies! First, tell me why you're here!!
Tone my abs.
Cardio workout.
Lose those last 5 lbs.
Um, I wanted to get out of the house...
weirdo
To be honest, I had also hoped to make a mom friend.
But after my zillionth set of lunges, it was starting to feel like a mistake.
Then came the instructor's next announcement...
We're running next class, so if you have a newborn, definitely wear a pad because I guarantee you'll leak!!!

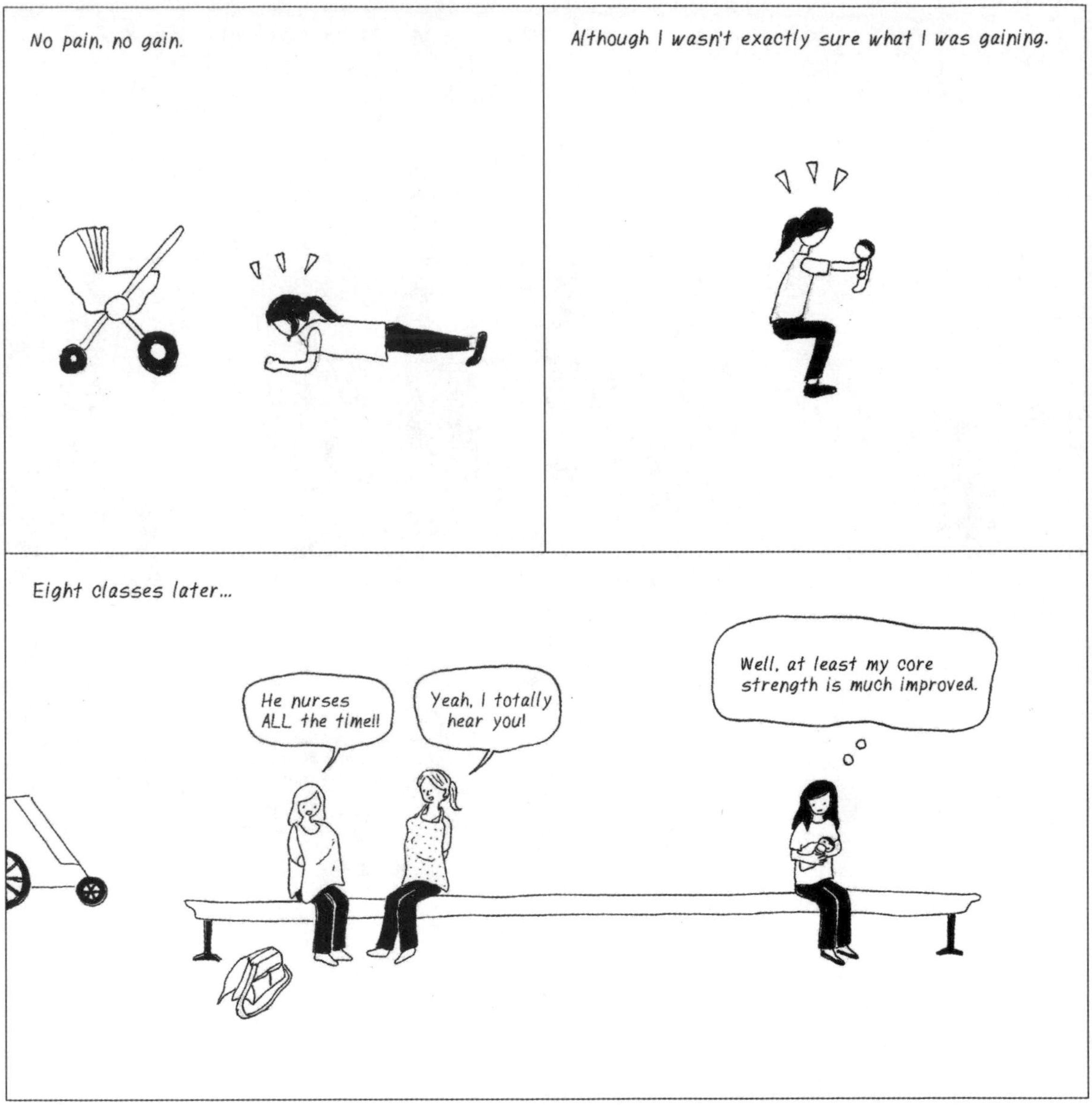
No pain, no gain.
Although I wasn't exactly sure what I was gaining.
Eight classes later...
He nurses ALL the time!!
Yeah, I totally hear you!
Well, at least my core strength is much improved.

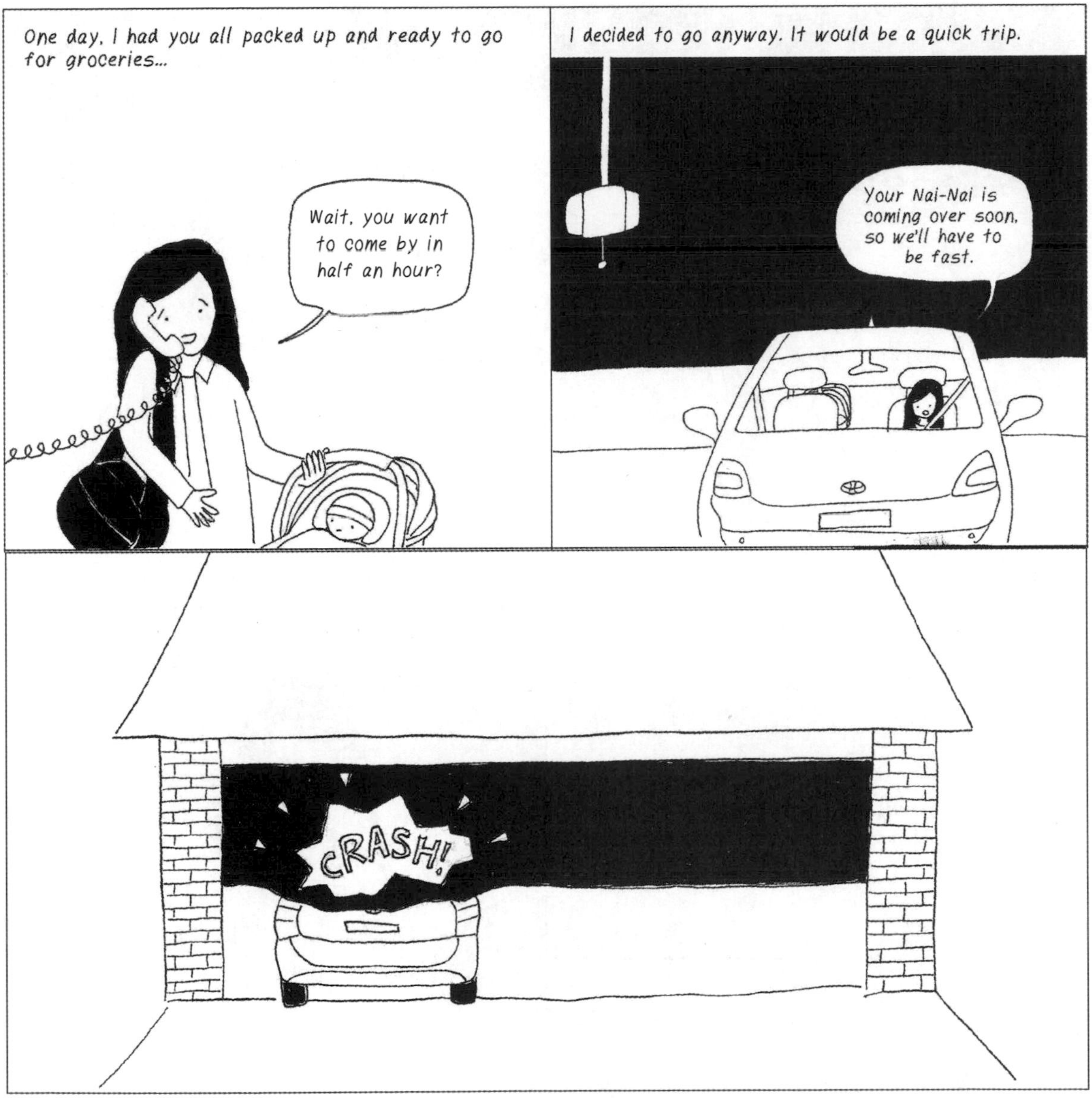
One day, I had you all packed up and ready to go for groceries...
Wait, you want to come by in half an hour?
I decided to go anyway. It would be a quick trip.
Your Nai-Nai is coming over soon, so we'll have to be fast.
CRASH!

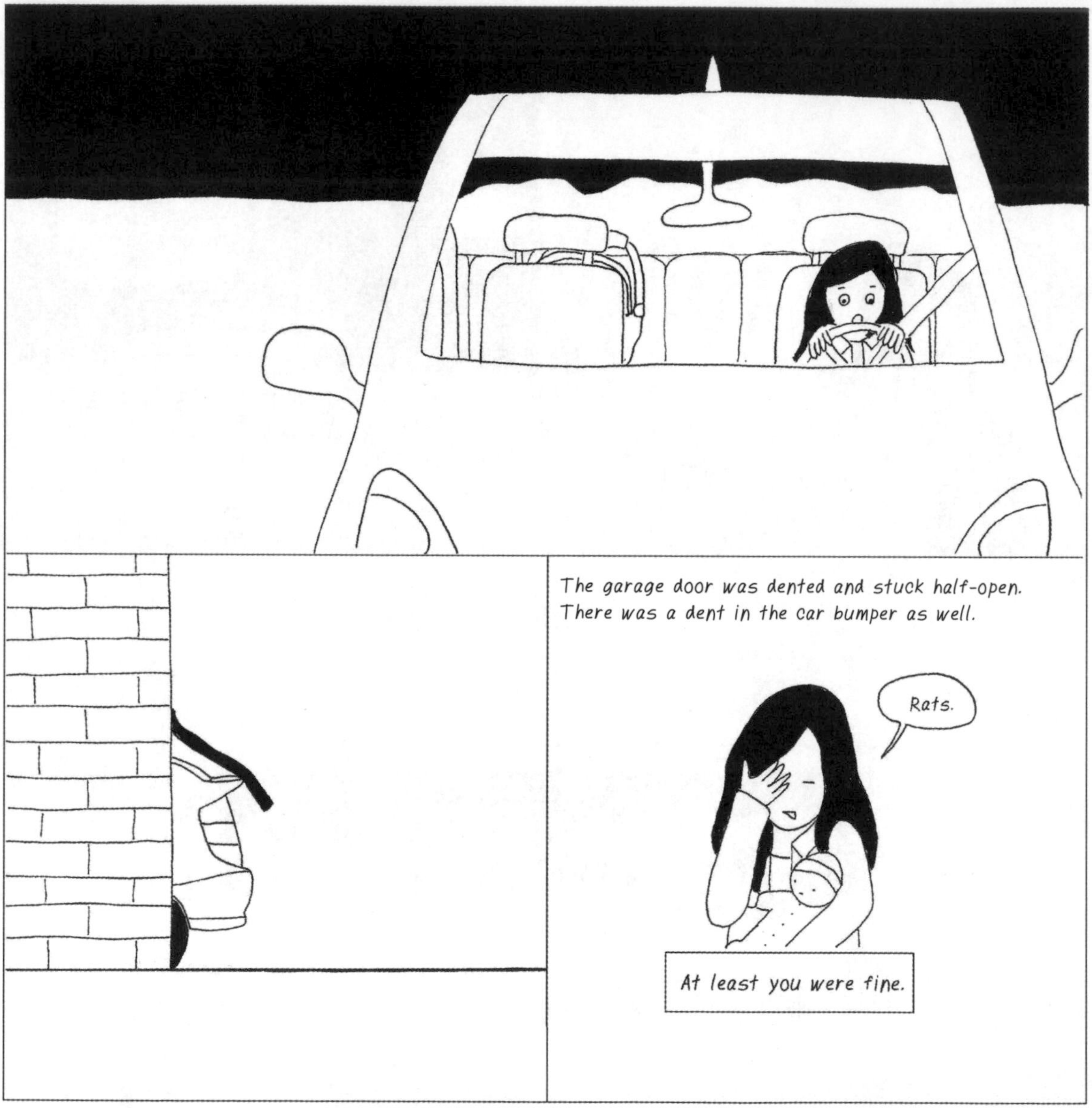
The garage door was dented and stuck half-open.
There was a dent in the car bumper as well.
Rats.
At least you were fine.

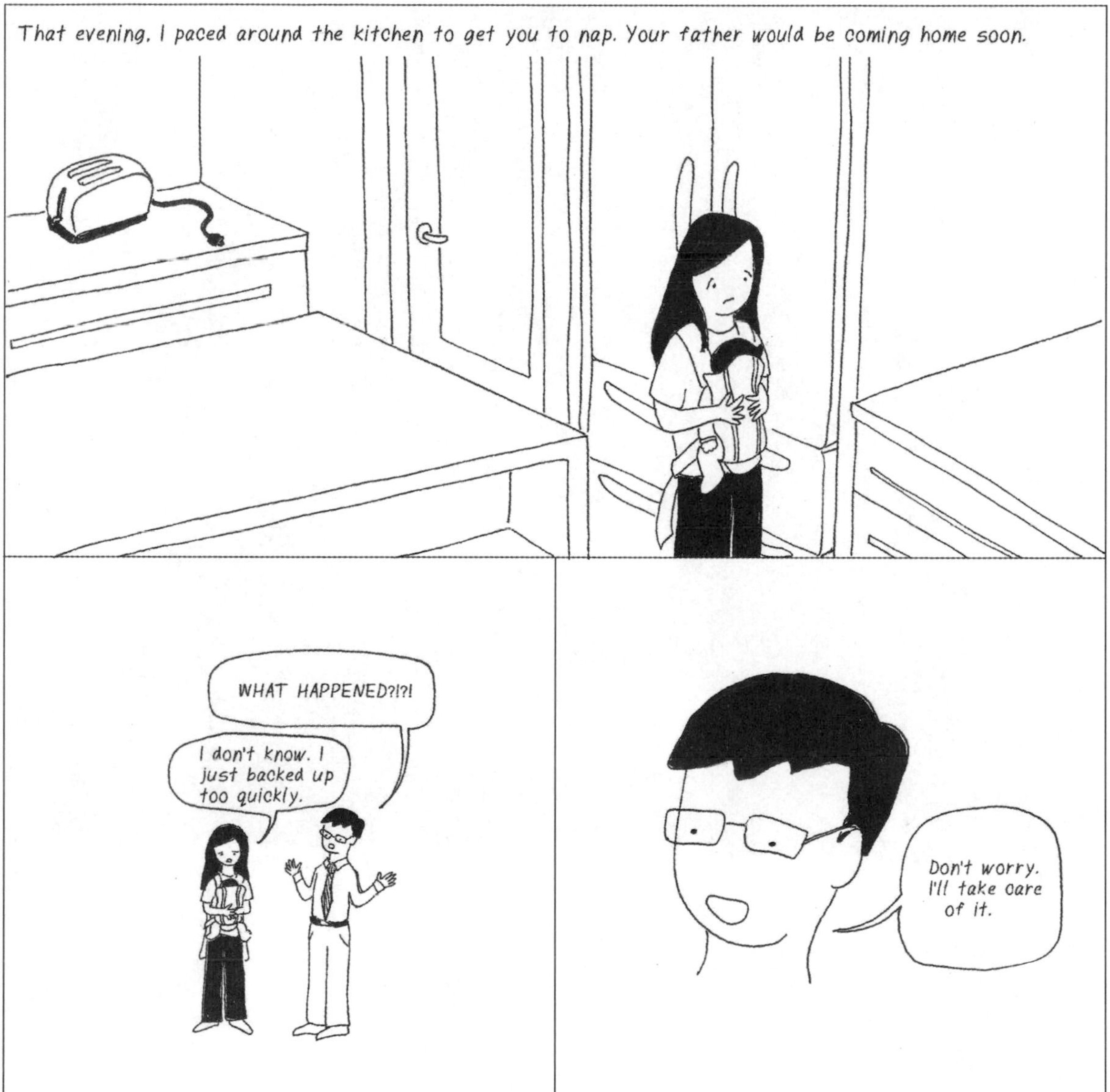
That evening, I paced around the kitchen to get you to nap. Your father would be coming home soon.
WHAT HAPPENED?!?!
I don't know. I just backed up too quickly.
Don't worry. I'll take care of it.

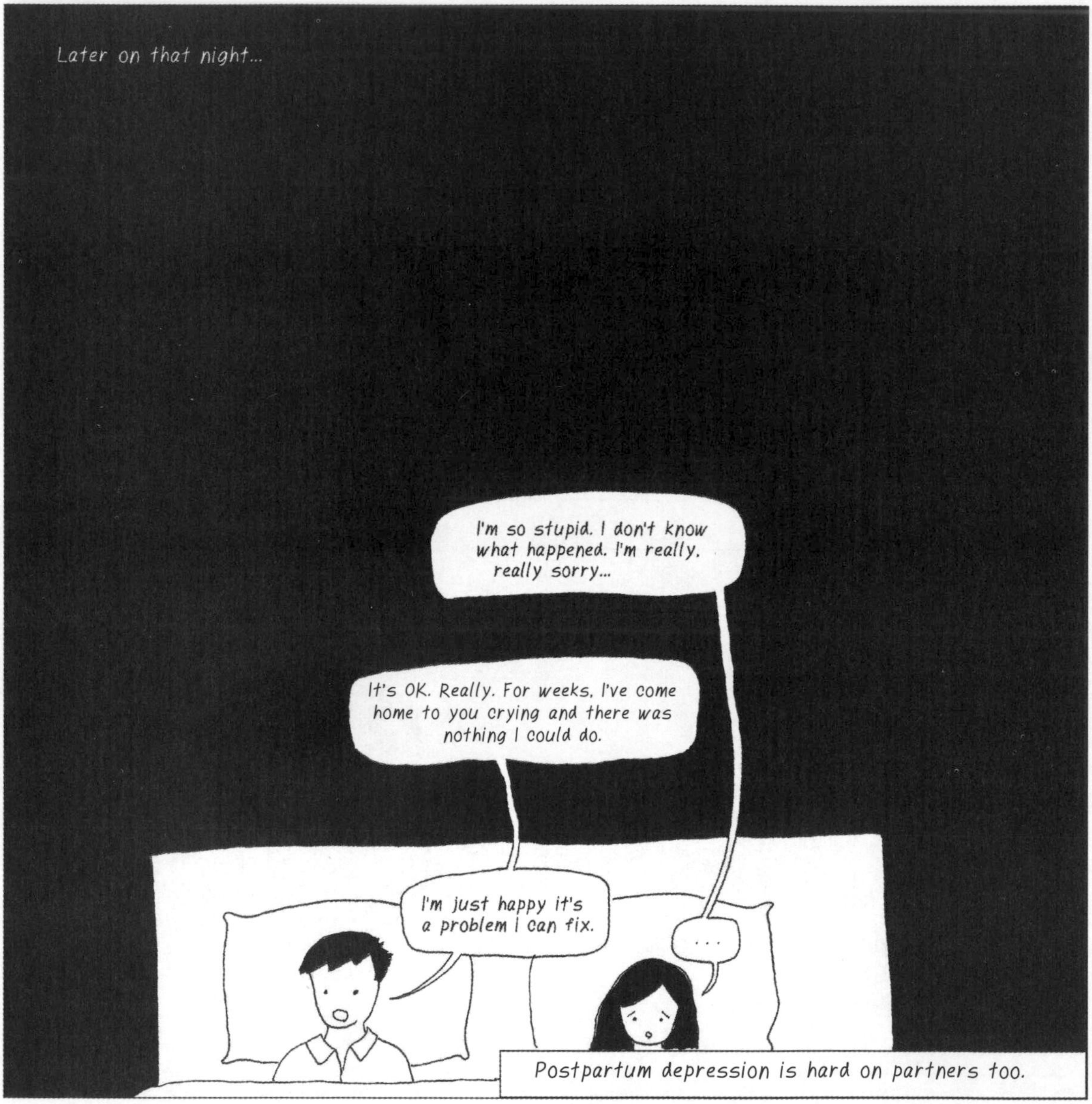
Later on that night...
I'm so stupid. I don't know what happened. I'm really, really sorry...
It's OK. Really. For weeks, I've come home to you crying and there was nothing I could do.
I'm just happy it's a problem I can fix.
. . .
Postpartum depression is hard on partners too.

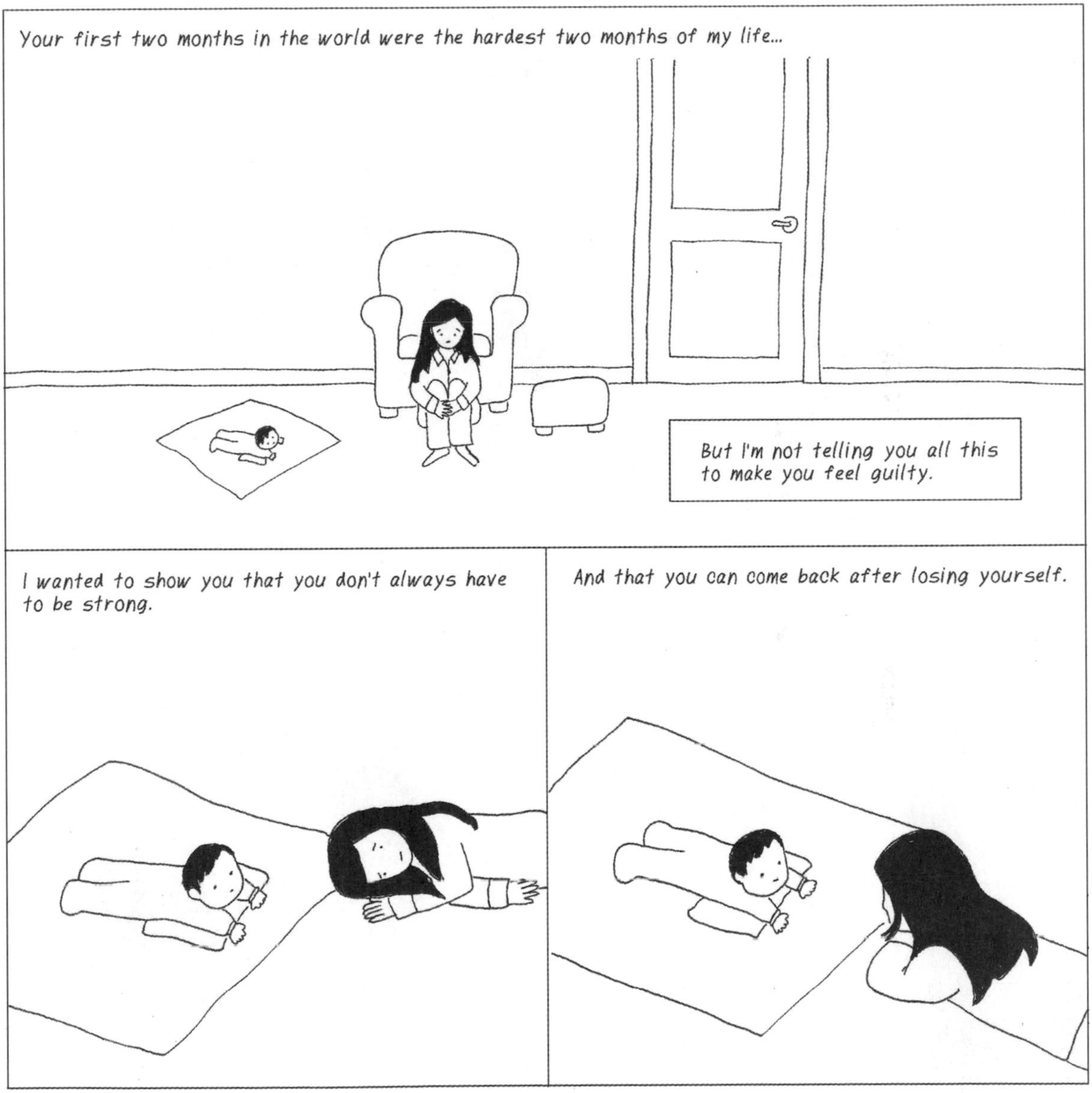
Your first two months in the world were the hardest two months of my life...
But I'm not telling you all this to make you feel guilty.
I wanted to show you that you don't always have to be strong.
And that you can come back after losing yourself.

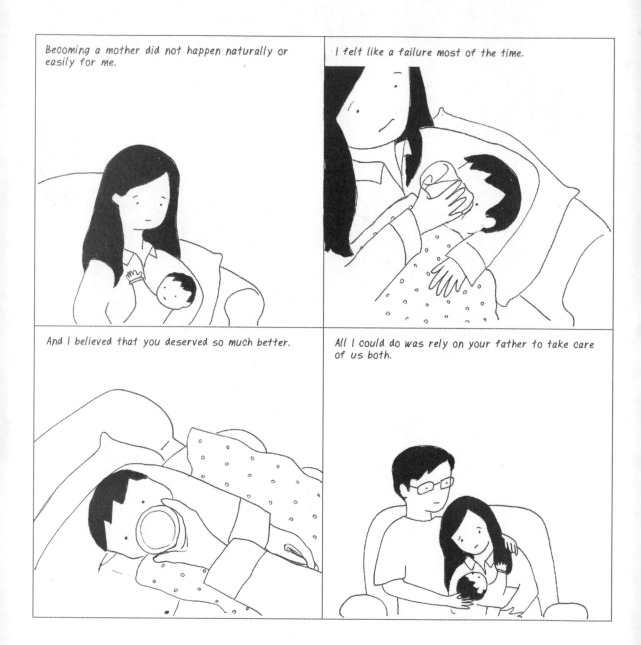

Becoming a mother did not happen naturally or easily for me.

I felt like a failure most of the time.

And I believed that you deserved so much better.

All I could do was rely on your father to take care of us both.

I wanted
to die, but
I'm thankful
I didn't.

I hope you never go through depression, postpartum or otherwise.

But if you do, please know that I know what it's like.

Rilke's advice was to remain still in the sadness, and to let it transform you into someone different.

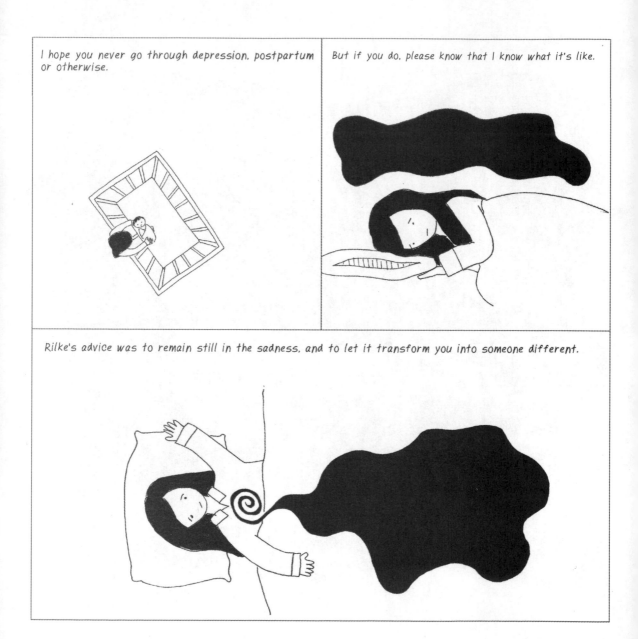

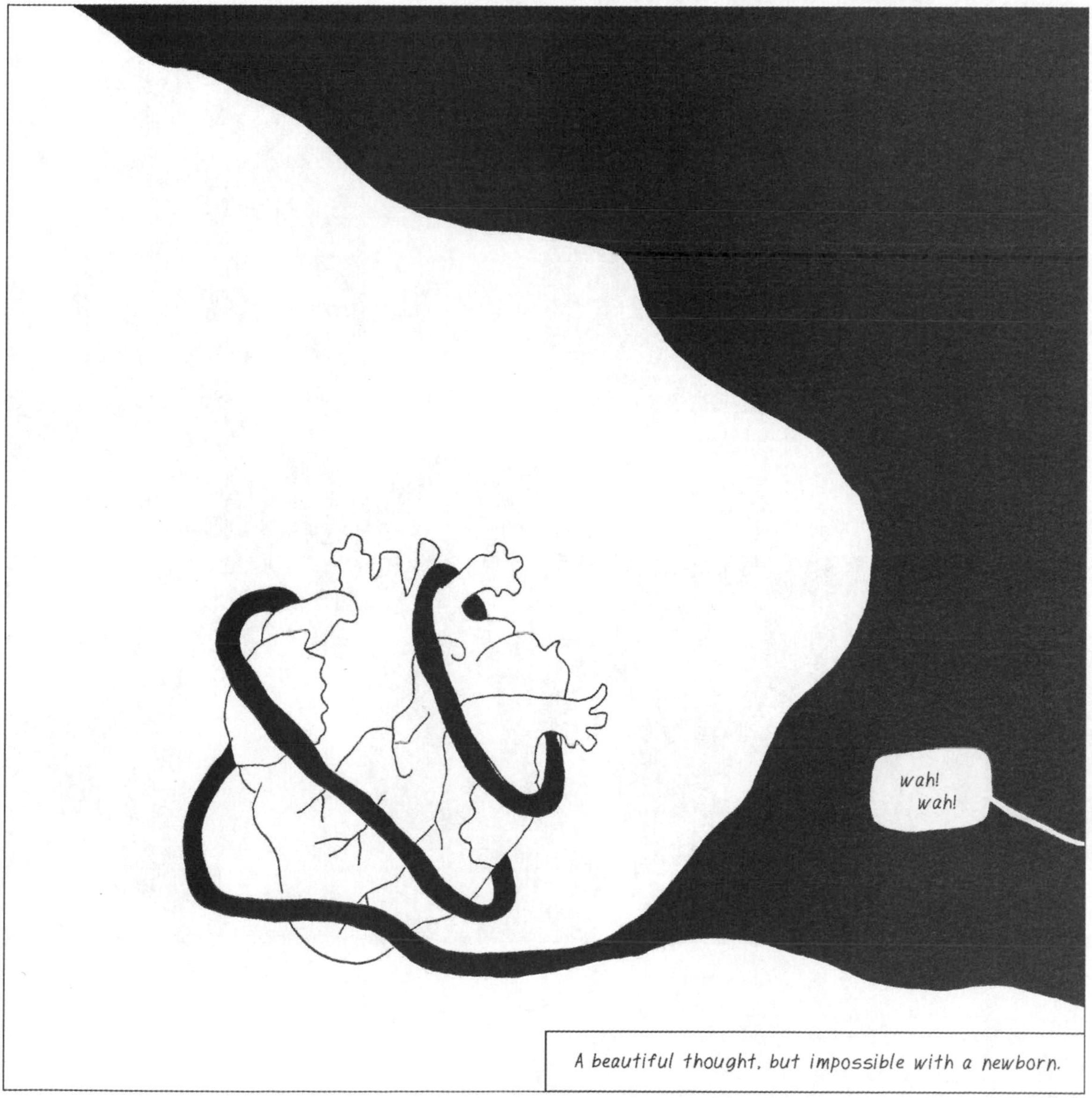
wah!
wah!
A beautiful thought, but impossible with a newborn.

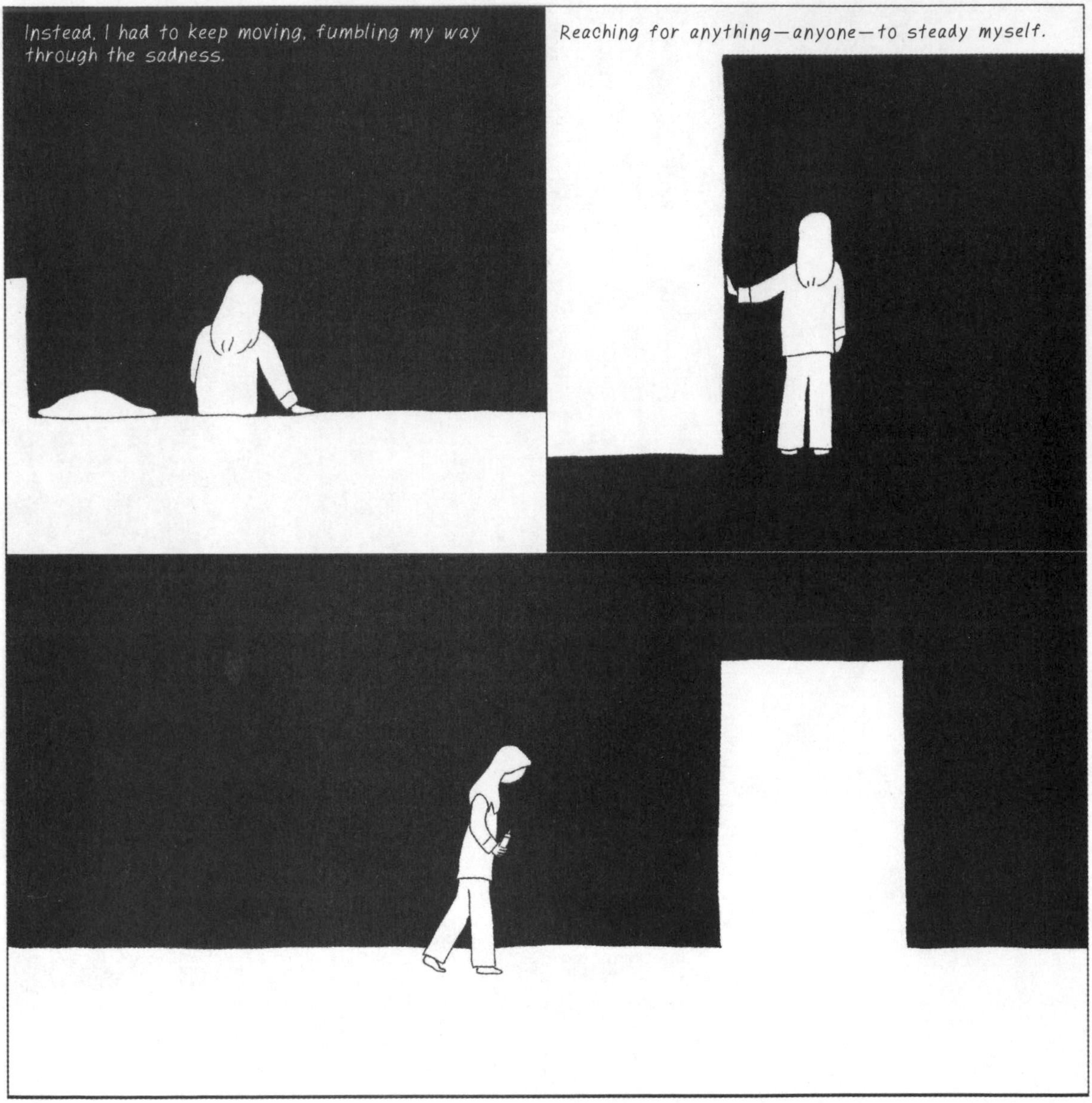
Instead, I had to keep moving, fumbling my way through the sadness.
Reaching for anything—anyone—to steady myself.

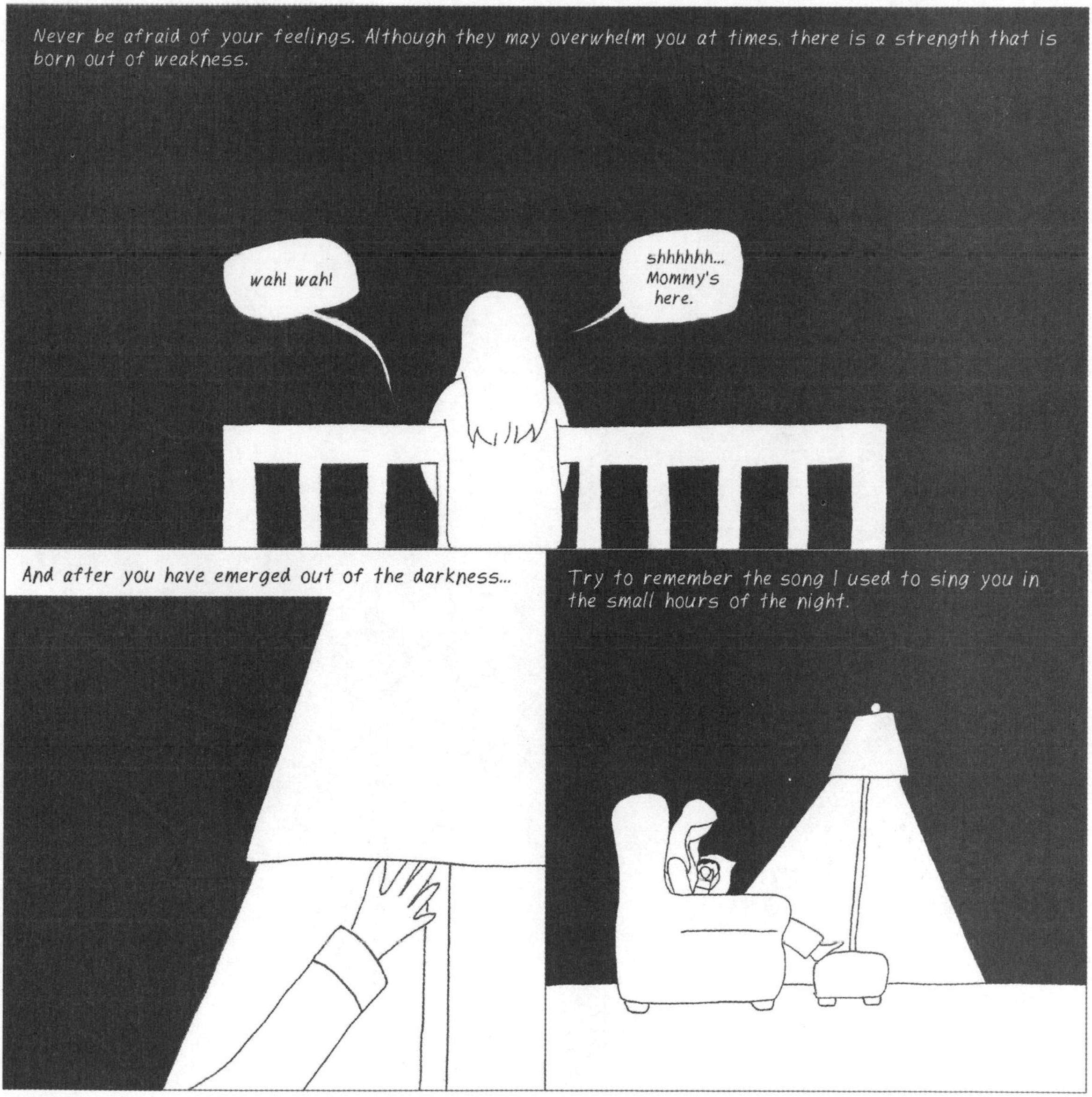
Never be afraid of your feelings. Although they may overwhelm you at times, there is a strength that is born out of weakness.
wah! wah!
shhhhhh... Mommy's here.
And after you have emerged out of the darkness...
Try to remember the song I used to sing you in the small hours of the night.

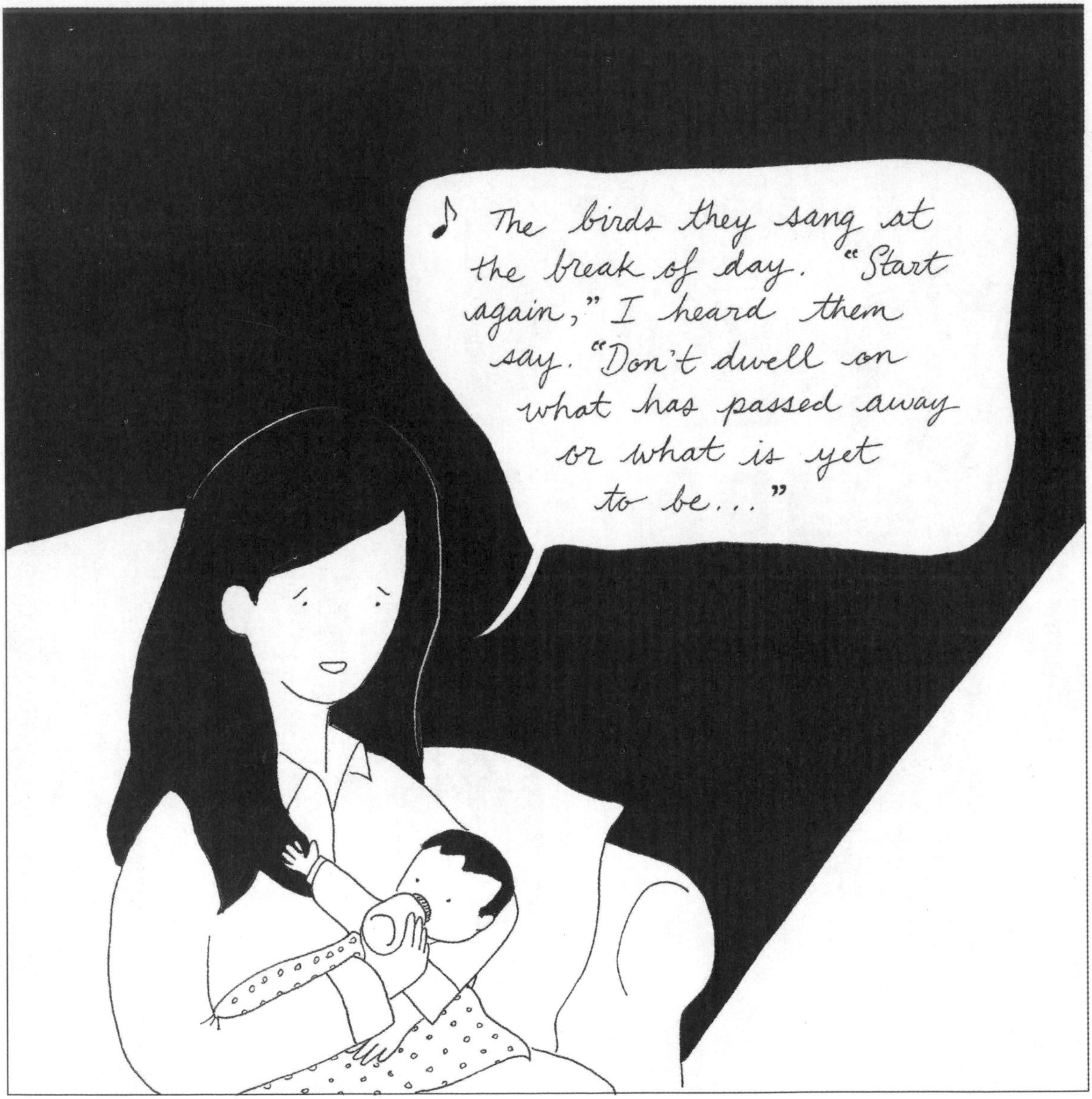
♪ The birds they sang at the break of day. "Start again," I heard them say. "Don't dwell on what has passed away or what is yet to be..."

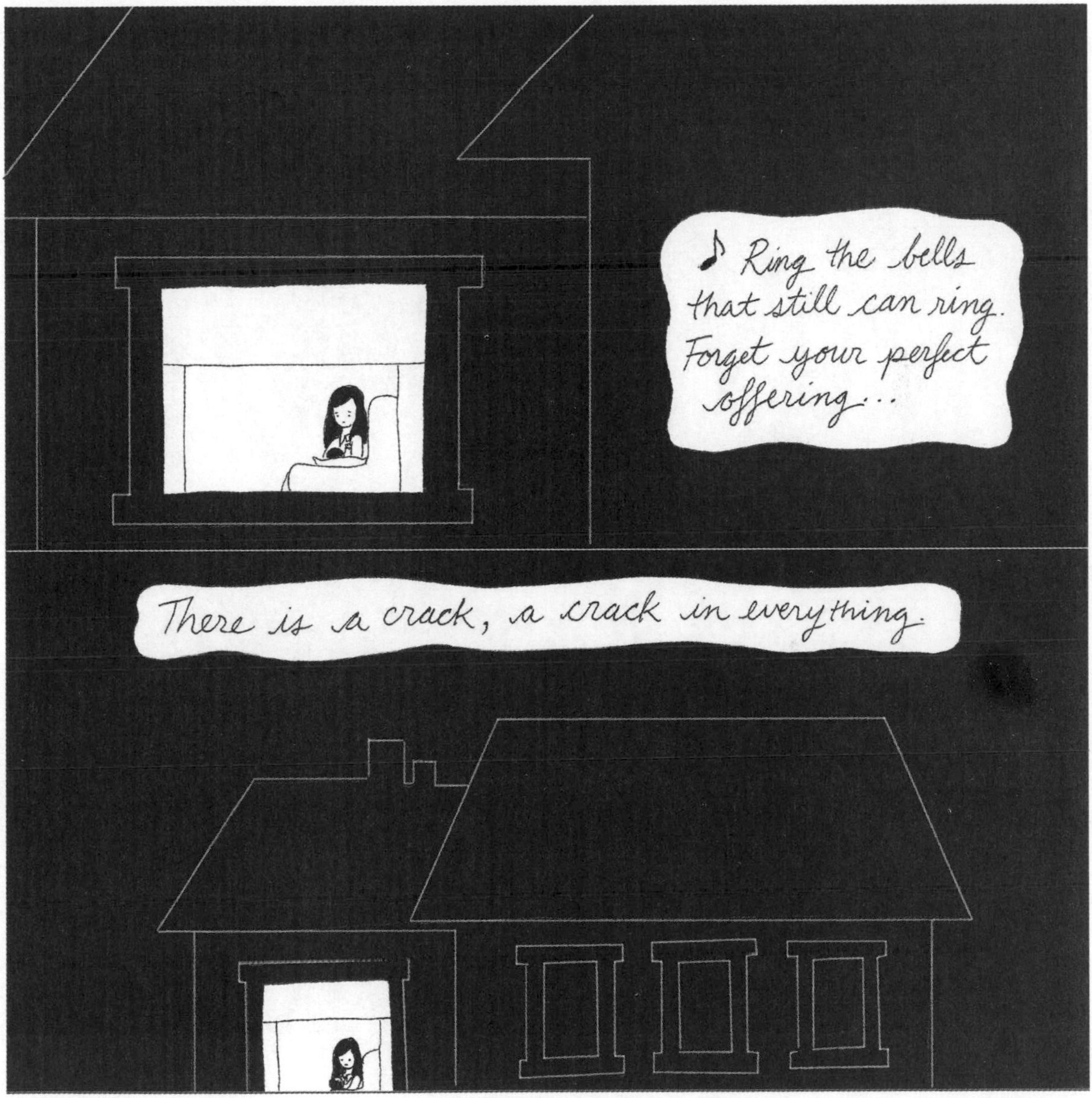
♪ Ring the bells that still can ring. Forget your perfect offering...
There is a crack, a crack in everything.

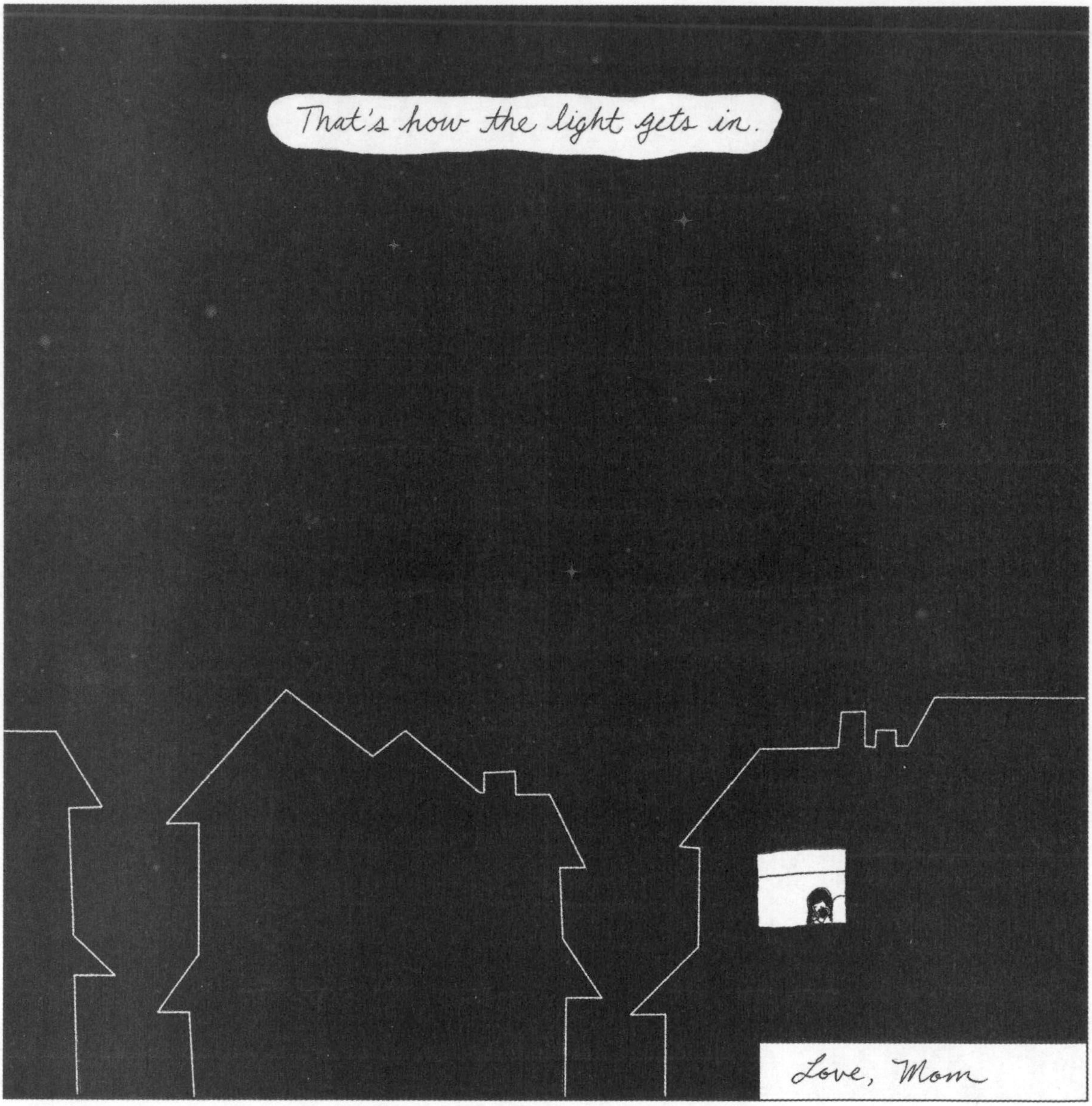
That's how the light gets in.
Love, Mom

Postscript

I wrapped up my weekly counselling sessions and stopped taking anti-depressants when Scarlet turned eight months old. A week later, I discovered I was pregnant with my second baby.

I was appalled at the prospect of having two kids under two—I could barely manage one under one—but also saw the new baby as a fresh start. I told myself it would be different this time.

Sunny decided to take six months off work, and my doula, AJ, planned to be with me starting in the delivery room. My mom offered to take Scarlet a few days a week to give me more rest.

I had an uncomplicated pregnancy, and a standard labour and delivery, which brought us a tiny, only slightly premature baby girl we named Eden. She was perfect. And although the first few months were a blur of breastfeeding, colic, gastro-esophageal reflux and bouncing on that stupid ball, it all felt manageable.

But soon after Sunny went back to work, the darkness returned. I was so disappointed in myself. I thought, *If I were stronger, this wouldn't be happening again.* Clearly, I was broken—too broken to be a good mother.

I remember going to pick up Eden's baby Zantac for her reflux one evening and listening to Stars' "Calendar Girl" as I drove home. The sun set over the foothills as I counted off months of the year along with the song:

> *January, February, March, April, May—I'm alive.*
> *June, July, August, September, October—I'm alive.*
> *November, December, yeah all through the winter—I'm alive.*
> *I'm alive.*

As the music swelled to a crescendo, I decided I had to stay alive. It would be my only goal for now, the only aspect of being a "good mother" I could achieve each day. I would stay alive for my girls.

My parents often use a Cantonese word—*ngai*—that seems, to me, more complete and compelling than the English word "endure." Although it contains the same idea of patient suffering as "endure," it goes further, acknowledging that difficulties are not unusual, and that often life is about waiting it out in a sort of joyless existence.

This approach may not be right for everyone with postpartum depression, but it's what I needed to get through the days until I found a new psychiatrist and began another course of treatment. I stayed alive. I *ngai.*

It was a vital shift in my thinking. Until then, I'd mistakenly thought my family would be better off without me, since I couldn't seem to do the things I was supposed to do. But if the only thing I needed to do was stay alive ... well, maybe.

So I did.

And the joy came later, after doing cognitive behavioural therapy and learning how to be kinder to myself. After I realized that I don't need to be a good mother—whatever that even means. I just need to be here.

Less than three years later, I found myself again with a newborn. Isaac came via speedy delivery, and I went home with him 24 hours later. That night, while nursing, I stroked his little head and felt a sudden flood of happiness and pride. The overwhelming sense of well-being caught me off guard, and I thought, *Oh, so this is what those other mothers were talking about!* It had only taken me three babies to get there.

Motherhood is intense. It is both wonderful and unbearable, often at the same time. And I don't believe there is only one right way to feel about it—just as there is no singular definition of a good mother—but I was grateful for that moment of peace nonetheless. There was hope for me yet.

Love,
Teresa

Acknowledgments

Thank you to the entire team at Arsenal Pulp Press—especially Brian Lam, Shirarose Wilensky and Oliver McPartlin—for taking a risk on a new author with a strangely hacked together manuscript about a topic most would rather avoid. I am inspired by your bold vision for Canadian literature and can only hope my voice adds something of value.

Thanks to my agent, Carly Watters, for helping me navigate the book world. And to the Binders for the same.

I am grateful to all the early readers of various drafts of this book, without whom I would've given up. In particular: Adele Brunnhofer, Susanne Evans, Dominic Fabrig, Karen Chu Gervais, John Hamilton, Doug Hironaka, Brynne Harding, Jeff Kubik, Karen McKinnon, Tara MacKinnon, Abby Miller, Monica Sommerville, Karen Styles and Narissa Tadros. Special thanks to Ginny Mulligan and Katrina Regino, for your graphic design talent (and also your friendship).

Mélanie LaPointe, *Dear Scarlet* is as much yours as it is mine. From helping me with revisions to supporting me through all the rejections, you have been this book's fiercest champion. *Merci de tout mon coeur.*

Thank you to Julie Wong, who sat at the table next to me while I pencilled and inked night after night, and turned what could've been an isolating endeavour into a time of healing for us both.

I'm also deeply indebted to those who supported me and my babies through postpartum depression and new motherhood: AJ Hadfield, Dr Lorraine Natho, my Northside family, Sene Tkaczuk, Michael and Hannah Ng, Stephen and Lily Wong and my parents, Frank and Mun Kam Ng.

Sunny Wong is the hero of this story and the love of my life. And to Scarlet, Eden and Isaac: I'm so grateful to be your mother. I love you, I love you, I love you.

Soli Deo gloria.

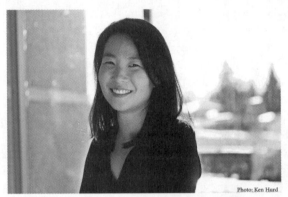

TERESA WONG is a Calgary writer who had three children in less than five years. At first, she feared motherhood would destroy her but is pleasantly surprised to find herself continually remade. When the kids are asleep, she writes and draws pictures. When she is asleep, it's never for long. *Dear Scarlet* is her first book.
byteresawong.com